GLUTEN-FREE
BREWING

TECHNIQUES, PROCESSES, AND INGREDIENTS
FOR CRAFTING FLAVORFUL BEER

T0015216

BY ROBERT KEIFER

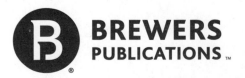

BREWERS
PUBLICATIONS™

Brewers Publications®
A Division of the Brewers Association
PO Box 1679, Boulder, Colorado 80306-1679
BrewersAssociation.org
BrewersPublications.com

Proudly Printed in the United States of America.
10 9 8 7 6 5 4 3 2 1
ISBN-13: 978-1-938469-75-6
ISBN-10: 1-938469-75-5
EISBN: 978-1-938469-76-3

Library of Congress Control Number: 2022940704

Publisher: Kristi Switzer
Technical Editor: Alan Windhausen
Copyediting: Iain Cox
Indexing: Doug Easton
Art Direction: Jason Smith
Interior Design & Production: Justin Petersen
Cover Photo © Aaron Colussi

Table of Contents

Acknowledgments

This book is an homage to all the gluten-free brewers that came before me, and who have freely shared their experiences in this space with brewers like me, and now you. Ancient grains are here to usher us into the next chapter of brewing, where a blending of new and old will create something never dreamt of before. I'm humbled by the opportunity to represent these grains, techniques and brewers in the same way my hero, Charlie Papazian, has represented homebrewing with barley.

Furthermore, I'd like to say a big thanks to Brewers Publications for its receptiveness to this topic specifically and for its quest to help people know everything there is to know about brewing in general. The shared passion behind brewing is something that grounds me and keeps me focused on making this a definitive guide on gluten-free brewing.

Of course, I would like to thank my wife for the all the incredible support she gave me in writing this book.

Introduction

NO BARLEY, NO WHEAT, NO RYE? NO PROBLEM!

You may be here for several reasons. Perhaps your doctor recommended removing gluten from your diet for a medical condition, for example, celiac disease, a wheat or barley allergy, irritable bowel syndrome (IBS), Hashimoto's thyroiditis, ataxia, or non-celiac gluten sensitivity (NCGS). You could be an experienced home or commercial brewer interested in expanding your brewing repertoire and knowledge beyond barley-based beer. Maybe you are looking to expand your beer lineup and safely meet the needs of gluten-free consumers. Finally, perhaps someone you care about has been forced to or chosen to limit or eliminate dietary gluten and you want to help them enjoy a beer again. Depending on where you are in the world, homebrewing may be your only option for consuming gluten-free beer.

The focus on barley in brewing, and the hundreds of years of research that has gone into using barley for this purpose, has had a deep and lasting impact on the world of beer. But what did brewers do in parts of the world where barley did not (yet) exist or had not yet become the chief "beer-making" grain? They used whatever they had on hand. The Incas, Mayans, sub-Saharan African cultures, and those throughout Asia—these peoples were making grain-based non-barley beers for a long time, some as far back as 10,000 years ago or more. Many of these beverages are still consumed today. Yes, mead, wine, cider, and other fermented beverages have their place in brewing history, but what about *beer* made from grains other than barley?

When I started brewing without barley the internet age was in full swing, and many gluten-free brewing trailblazers had already done much of the legwork that forms the scientific backbone for this book. In just a short span of time—really in the decade from 2011 to 2021—gluten-free brewing has undergone some incredible leaps forward. A small cadre of maltsters has forged new techniques to deal with ancient grains and bring to market products that either previously did not exist or that required a ridiculous level of skill for most would-be gluten-free brewers. In that same time frame, a small number of craft brewers have begun to explore new brewing techniques and redefine the gluten-free beer market, which was previously dominated by just a few sorghum-based lagers, such as Lakefront's New Grist (released in 2005) and Anheuser-Busch's Redbridge (released 2006). Best of all, the gluten-free home-brewing community has begun to coalesce, sharing knowledge, collaborating on citizen science experiments, and generally pushing the envelope as homebrewers never miss an opportunity to tinker. We literally would not be here today with such amazing options for gluten-free drinkers without all the work that the community has put in.

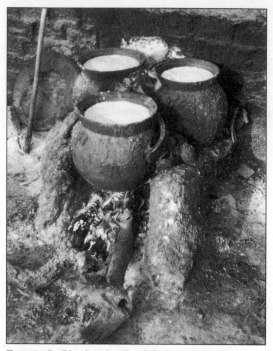

Figure 0.1. Traditional sorghum beer being brewed in a sub-Saharan African village. Traditional sorghum beers go by many names depending on where you are in Africa, for example, *bil-bil* in Cameroon, *omalovu* in Namibia, *umqombothi* in Zambia and some parts of South Africa, and *pombe* across East Africa, and many more names besides. Evidence for beers like these date as far back as the Bronze Age in sub-Saharan Africa, which could mean they were being made as long ago as 2300 BCE. © *Getty/Robert Ford*

And yet, there is still some distance to cover before gluten-free brewing becomes as established and accessible as "conventional" (barley-based) brewing. Beyond obvious cases where there is a medical reason to avoid gluten, consumers and brewing industry members may struggle to put gluten-free beer in context: is it a method, a style, or simply a fad?

Celiac disease has likely been around since the Agricultural Revolution (Gasbarrini et. al. 2014, 255), and with no realistic "cure" on the horizon it is certainly not a fad.[1] A style suggests a reasonably narrow set of codified parameters. While the obvious parameter is ingredients, other parameters include alcoholic strength, flavor and aroma elements, and appearance. Gluten-free beer can run the gamut of conventional (and unusual) beer styles, from delicate, highly drinkable lagers to complex imperial stouts and mixed-culture saisons and sours.

In this book, my goal is to demonstrate that gluten-free brewing is an *approach* that is not simply defined by what it omits (barley, wheat, and rye) but more so by the ingredients it includes. These are ingredients that span continents and millennia, and are continually being adapted through the innovations of maltsters, brewers, and scientists.

Use this as a how-to book to understand the various grains now available to brewers, some that mimic their gluten-containing cousins and some that bring new complexity to certain beer styles. Once you understand the flavors that they elicit, you will also come to realize that these grains have the potential to create new styles entirely.

For some, this book may be an interesting armchair foray into a weird, parallel brewing universe. For others, it may point to the only real path to reclaiming an otherwise off-limits beverage. Who knows, you may be just one diagnosis away from becoming an exclusively gluten-free beer drinker yourself.

---

[1]   In fact, there is a clinical report of this ailment from as early as 250 CE (Gasbarrini et al. 2014, 251).

The world of beer is undergoing a renaissance due to the rise of craft brewing, and consumers are no longer content with mass-market appeal. This taste revolution came about because drinkers learned to trust the little guys with open minds and willing palates. Today, the business plans of up-and-coming breweries and brands often have a specific niche in mind, which has caused so much innovation in the past decade that at least one new Beer Judge Certification Program (BJCP) beer style has been added each year. This new buzz is everything beer has always promised to be and then some, and it is only getting better. That is especially true in gluten-free brewing, which is a niche of a niche of a niche.

I remember being 22 and discovering I was intolerant to gluten . . . It could not have come at a worse time as I had just discovered craft beer. The journey for many, depending on where and when you go gluten free, can be quite depressing. Even today there are very few beers made without barley and wheat. I was basically fated to become a homebrewer, and this book for the most part represents my and other brewers' experience with brewing gluten free up to this point.

GLUTEN-FREE BREWING TODAY

The growth and success of gluten-free brewing is owed almost exclusively to homebrewers, maybe like yourself, who have helped push this space forward. Many of the gluten-free breweries open today were founded by homebrewers going pro. Gluten-free brewing will need the ingenuity of homebrewers if it is to become a staple of the modern craft beer scene. Remember, you are not alone—there are thousands (dare I say, millions) of people that are brewing naturally gluten-free beers, and in some cultures have been doing so for thousands of years.

Since making the decision to brew 100% gluten-free beer, many things have happened for me. I became one of the founding members of the Zero Tolerance Gluten Free Homebrew Club (https://zerotolerance.mywikis.net/), which has since grown to over 1,500 member brewers spread over

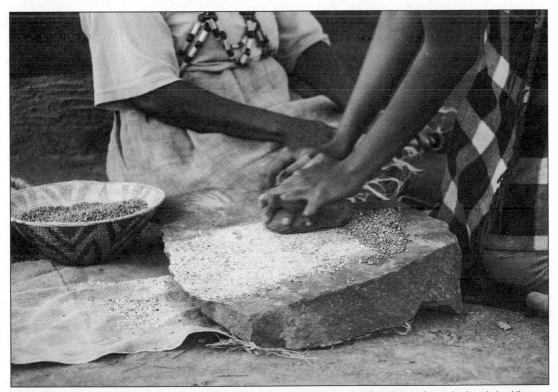

Figure 0.2. Traditional malt hand-grinding in Botswana. The grain shown is either sorghum or millet. Villagers often gather in a circle while grinding, singing various traditional songs. A porous stone is pushed back and forth on a smooth stone, which mimics the mechanical action of a roller in a grain mill. © Getty/poco_bw

five continents. The variety of styles and brewing techniques that have arisen from this group has helped create such a massive amount of growth in our space in just the few years since the club was formed in 2018. From competitions to hosting monthly meetings with industry guests, the club is arguably one of the most active and innovative remote-based homebrewing communities out there. I would contend that this is because much of gluten-free brewing has yet to be codified for the average entry-level brewer. It was writing this book that prompted much of the effort to collect the data that are represented in this book. Another thing that happened for me is that I also went pro, founding Divine Science Brewing with my wife (https://divinesciencebrewing.com).

In the chapters that follow, I will be comparing various home and professional brewers' recipe formulations and brewing techniques—particularly mashing—to help create what the gluten-free brewing community feels are true-to-style gluten-free beers. Many of these beers will taste the same as their barley-based cousins, whereas some are what could be called true-to-style millet beers, sorghum beers, rice beers, and maize beers (like *chicha*), which are very different to their barley-based relatives.

Any reader who has judged entries in the gluten-free category knows that this part of any competition is likely one of the hardest to assess at the commercial level, since this category can pit, say, imperial millet wines, saisons, lagers, and IPAs against one another. My premonition is that adding new, separate gluten-free styles will become necessary as more and more commercial brewers utilize these alternative grains. For homebrewers it is even more testing, since gluten-free homebrewers have to

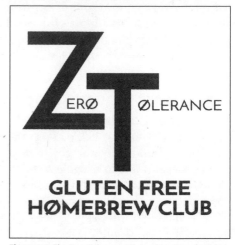

Figure 0.3. The Zero Tolerance Gluten Free Homebrewing Club wiki and Facebook pages are a treasure trove for gluten-free brewers, with recipes, techniques, and in-depth discussions about all things gluten free. *Art courtesy of Cale Baldwin.*

compete in the Alternative Grain Beer category (31a), in which beers containing barley and wheat can compete so long as they contain "non-standard brewing grains . . . added or used exclusively." In this case, spelt (a wheat variety) and rye count as non-standard. Adjusting the BJCP guidelines to include a dedicated gluten-free category seems necessary at this time, and would bring the BJCP in line with commercial competitions such as the World Beer Cup® and the Great American Beer Festival® (GABF™).

BACK TO THE FUTURE

Gluten-free brewing is not just a contemporary phenomenon, it is very much brewing's past as well. Styles like chicha (Incan corn beer) and the polyonymous African sorghum beer date back over 10,000 years and are still drunk today by people in their respective native cultures. The societal impact of these beers can still be seen throughout many present-day community gatherings and religious ceremonies that involve group drinking. You can watch YouTube videos from modern-day Namibia where a sorghum mash is stirred with a palm frond and fermented in a clay pot underground—ancient methods that have served an incredibly foundational purpose and show their purpose still today. And who can forget Sam Calagione's televised foray into chicha, spitting chewed corn into a bowl?[2] Brewing with these ancient ingredients (with a modern twist most times) has opened my mind to things I would not otherwise have thought to try. I hope these ingredients find prominence in the current beer renaissance in the way that they truly deserve.

Practically an infant in the grain community, modern-day barley is a descendant of

---

2   *Brew Masters*, episode 2, "Chicha," directed by Bengt Anderson, featuring Sam Calagione, aired November 28, 2010, on Discovery Channel.

its mother strain, called *akiti*, which was cultivated about 10,000 years ago in the Fertile Crescent (ancient Mesopotamia) along with grains like einkorn (now called wheat); from there, barley made its way through northern Africa and much of Europe. Barley is now cultivated throughout the world (Cooper 2015). From there many have come to know the story, where barley was found not only to be a great foodstuff but also an incredible ingredient for making beer.

Today, while barley is still an important food crop, it is corn (maize), rice, and wheat that are the top three staple crops (in descending order) in terms of overall world production. In the modern era, the use of alternative grains and pseudocereals like millet, sorghum, and quinoa shifted more to livestock and bird feed, being grown as cover crops and for forage; but these crops have not been completely forgotten, as their increasing inclusion in modern Western diets attests. However, while you may see corn, rice, sorghum, or quinoa on your plate, they are not typically in your glass, at least, not beyond a minor adjunct role.

As modern globalization marches on, many ancient beer styles still existing around the world are falling under siege from large brewing conglomerates. In practice, many of the tactics used in the global brewing industry have been quite predatory, ripe with hostile takeovers: I am specifically talking about the history of sorghum beers in South Africa. The *New York Times* and various other publications have told the story of black-owned National Sorghum Breweries.[3] The Age of Imperialism witnessed an exportation of Western culture and ideals, including the imperialistic nations' drink of choice. Since most imperial powers of the modern era were European countries, globalization has been one of the best things for barley-based beer but not so much for local beverages and native cultures, as we have come to learn. I hope this book serves as a potential jumping-off point for you to explore cultures from the recent and distant past, and as a demonstration that beer is so much more than the prevailing Eurocentric view of styles and ingredients. But I also hope to show off the versatility of gluten-free grains and how you can use them to create world-class beer even within conventional rules to achieve beers that many cannot tell are gluten free.

PULQUE

While the story of globalization often focuses on Western hegemony over regions of Asia and Africa, we should not forget its effects on indigenous cultures of Central and South America as well. Having traveled to Central America, I can attest to the difficulty I faced when trying to find *pulque* (or "agave beer"), which is an alcoholic drink fermented from 10–12-year-old maguey. In speaking with certain restaurants that carried this drink, once they got over the shock of a gringo asking for what they called "a poor man's drink," they told me that their recipe was passed down through the generations and that the drink is almost extinct where they are from. Although pulque can be mixed with various ingredients like fruits, spices, and nuts, I prefer it straight up—it has a lovely balance of tart and sweet, with a strong aloe-like viscosity that belies an otherwise light and drinkable beverage. I hope products like "ranch waters"[4] are a prelude to pulque's epic North and Central American comeback!

Gluten-free ingredients are being researched more than they ever were, and various desirable brewing characteristics within these grains are becoming better understood with each passing year. Yet, at this point in our understanding, there is almost no wrong way to use these grains, specifically because every beer recipe done in this space can be used as a data point (although I have found a couple of ways not to do it, as you will see in the coming chapters). In fact, many of the data points presented in this book come from homebrewers and commercial brewers just

---

[3] Donald G. McNeil Jr., "Not Thriving in Its Homeland;Beer Disappoints as Black South African Business," *New York Times*, October 3, 1995, sec. D, p. 1, National edition, https://www.nytimes.com/1995/10/03/business/not-thriving-in-its-homeland-beer-disappoints-as-black-south-african-business.html.

[4] A tequila cocktail that features sparkling water, lime juice, and tequila.

like you. I invite *you* to participate in our ongoing research of these gluten-free grains and beer recipes—our collective understanding grows with each successive brew.

ABOUT THE BOOK

Chapter 1 will go over the nature of gluten and how it relates to celiac disease, and briefly discuss what constitutes truly gluten-free beer; chapter 2 will discuss where to find ingredients with which to brew such beer and general considerations when deciding what ingredients to use. Chapter 3 will be an exploration of various gluten-free base malts, character malts, and adjuncts that are currently available. Chapter 4 will get into recipe formulation through the lens of barley-based beer styles that are popular or lend themselves well to gluten-free versions. Chapter 5 concludes the first part of the book and is an in-depth look at brewing techniques to achieve any style. A section of recipe chapters for gluten-free beers follows, broadly grouped by geographical and/or cultural regions and the styles they are known for.

This book aims far beyond making something that is simply palatable. Through the course of trying the recipes you will find in this book and those you will create on your own, I am confident that you will notice the incredible flavors you can elicit from the not-so-new cornucopia of ingredients available. Some might make you altogether forget about conventional conceptions of how beer should taste. This book is about brewing full-flavored gluten-free beer and creating recipes that can be brewed for barley-dominated competitions and stand on their own as world-class beers. Cheers!

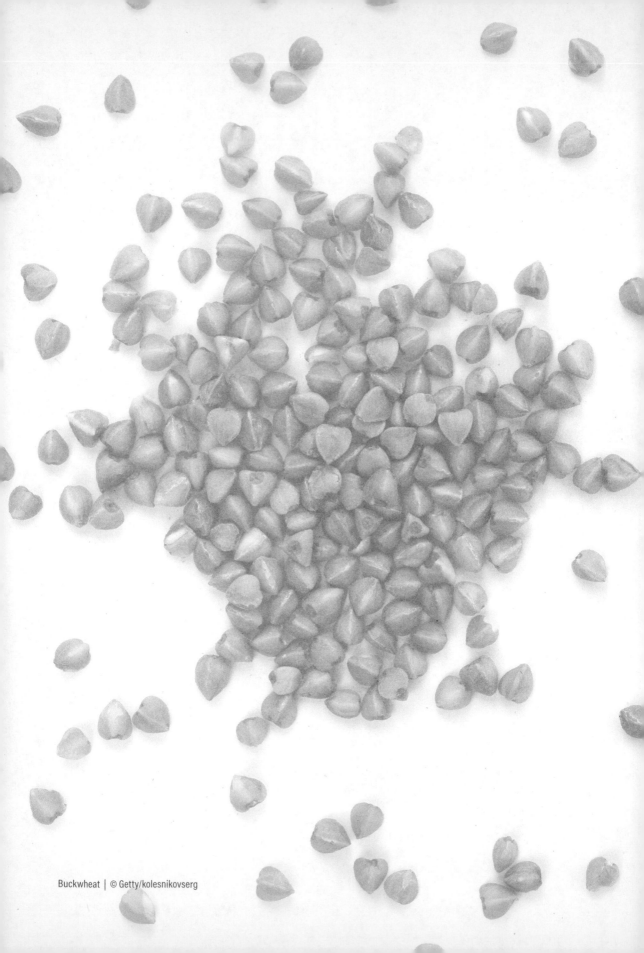

Buckwheat | © Getty/kolesnikovserg

1
Gluten:
A Multifaceted View

WHAT IS GLUTEN?

G*luten* is really more of a catch-all term. It describes a specific group of closely related but distinct proteins found in specific grasses, or cereals. While technically gluten refers to the complex protein structure that functions as a seed storage protein (mainly a nitrogen reserve) in wheat kernels (grains), a number of evolutionarily, structurally, and functionally similar proteins found in other grains are also referred to as "gluten," though their scientific names differ. In wheat, gluten consists primarily of *gliadin* and *glutenin*, which are two different groups (or "families") of proteins that conglomerate together in the starchy endosperm of the grain, this overall conglomeration being gluten. Other major cereals that contain some form of gluten are barley (various *hordeins* being the equivalent of wheat gliadins and glutenins), rye (made up of various *secalins*), and oats (*avenins*, which are the oat equivalent of gliadins; oats do not have an equivalent of glutenin). The "gliadin-like" proteins in these cereals all fall under the broader class of *prolamin* storage proteins, and the "glutenin-like" proteins under the class of *glutelin* storage proteins. While there is not as clear of a link for glutelins, it is unequivocal that dietary prolamin—and by extension dietary gluten—from these grains triggers the immune response that causes celiac disease (Wieser, Koehler, and Konitzer 2014, 130–139).

People with celiac disease react to ingested gluten in its various forms as outlined above. For the purposes of this book, any time I refer to *gluten*, I am including all these various triggering prolamin and glutelin proteins that are expressed in wheat, barley, rye, their hybrids, and close relatives, which includes einkorn, emmer, spelt, and durum. It should also be noted that this discussion of gluten includes these various proteins in their entirety, as well as the smaller chains of amino acids (peptides) that gluten is digested into when consumed (amino acids are the building blocks of proteins). In fact, it is these smaller peptides that people with celiac disease react to after ingesting gluten, rather than the gluten complex as a whole.

For those with celiac disease (both asymptomatic and symptomatic), these proteins and their building blocks can do all sorts of things to the body. Most commonly, gluten-derived peptides are absorbed through the gut lining, primarily the small intestine, in a way that exposes immune cells of the digestive tract to the peptides and triggers an immune response (Wieser, Koehler, and Konitzer 2014, 49). There are hundreds of different peptide sequences that can cause a reaction in a person with celiac disease, with symptoms ranging from mild to acute (Cebolla et al. 2018).

A GLUTEN BY ANY OTHER NAME . . .

I have seen people get confused by the scientific nomenclature, to the point where they think that a 100% barley beer is safe for them since it does not contain wheat. While *gluten* can refer to the specific protein in wheat, in a dietary sense it includes an entire family of proteins, as outlined in table 1.1.

Table 1.1. Prolamins and glutelins in various grains

Group	Wheat	Rye	Barley
HMW	HMW-GS	HMW-secalins	D-hordeins
MMW	ω1,2-gliadins ω5-gliadins	ω-secalins -	C-hordeins -
LMW	LMW-GS γ-gliadins α-gliadins	γ-75k-secalins γ-40k-secalins -	B-hordeins γ-hordeins -

GS, glutenin subunits; HMW, high-molecular-weight; MMW, medium-molecular weight; LMW, low-molecular-weight.

> *Anyone who has brewed with barley has seen the large amounts of gluten-laden dust the milling process can create. But gluten can appear in a number of surprising places, anywhere from the dust on a stick of chewing gum to the sealant used on a wine barrel (many barrels are sealed with wheat paste), or even in skin lotion and shampoo.*

WHAT IS CELIAC DISEASE?

Celiac disease is a serious autoimmune disease that occurs in genetically predisposed people where the ingestion of gluten leads to damage in the small intestine.[1] For someone with celiac disease, navigating the world takes a considerable amount of reading labels and contacting manufacturers to ensure that a product neither contains nor is cross-contaminated with gluten. There are serious reasons for this concern—the proteins in gluten and their derivatives cause lesions in the gut, leading to inflammation of the gut lining and damage to the small intestine, as well as other symptoms that can manifest outside of the gastrointestinal system (Popp and Mäki 2019).

In celiac disease, the body reacts to gluten-derived peptides by mounting an immune response in various ways, which results in the classic symptoms of inflammation of the gut lining, villous atrophy (the death of cellular structures in the small intestine associated with food absorption), and increased gut permeability. Celiac disease is one of the most common autoimmune gastrointestinal diseases, affecting at least 0.5%–1.0% of the world's population (Caio et al. 2019, 2), which is around 80 million people, about the same as the population of Germany. A number of people are also

[1] "What is Celiac Disease?" Celiac Disease Foundation, accessed January 4, 2022, https://celiac.org/about-celiac-disease/what-is-celiac-disease/.

assumed to be undiagnosed, underdiagnosed, or misdiagnosed, so the truth could be that this disease is more widespread (Kowalski et al. 2017).

It is estimated that 70% of cases of celiac disease present with atypical symptoms that make differential diagnosis much more difficult; this means that many people who are experiencing symptoms because they have celiac disease may not receive a quick or accurate diagnosis and therefore do not know they are reacting to dietary gluten (Lucia et al. 2018). Gluten consumption has also been tied to many other symptoms besides inflammation, including irritable bowel syndrome (IBS), diabetes mellitus type I, severe hypoglycemia in diabetes mellitus type I, psoriasis, sleep apnea in children, neoplasia, atopic dermatitis, depression, subclinical synovitis in children, autism, and schizophrenia (Pruimboom and de Punder 2015, 1–2).

This also does not include other disorders or diseases that may benefit from a gluten-free diet, such as Hashimoto's thyroiditis, which affects over 14 million people in the US alone (Krysiak, Szkróbka, and Okopień 2019). There now seems to be a clinical link between Hashimoto's thyroiditis and intestinal permeability, which allows gluten, among other things, to enter the bloodstream and therefore cause harmful autoimmune responses like attacking the thyroid gland (Lerner, Jeremias, and Matthias 2017).

The extent of these extra-intestinal symptoms is just now becoming better understood. It is only in the past decade that asymptomatic celiac disease and non-celiac gluten sensitivity (NCGS) have been recognized as conditions by the medical community. This chapter will show that our understanding of gluten is dependent upon the available technology.

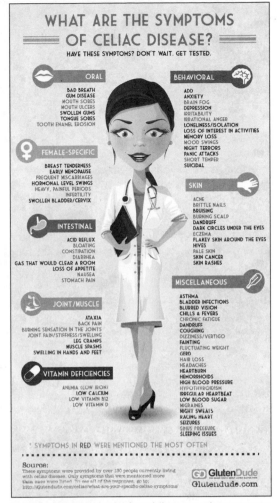

Fig 1.1. An infographic showing the varied symptoms that accompany celiac disease. *Courtesy of Gluten Dude, https://glutendude.com/what -are-celiac-disease-symptoms/.*

There is a joke in the gluten-free community: "How do you know you're talking to someone who's gluten free? Don't worry, they'll tell you . . ." It's true! I've caught myself suggesting people should go gluten free to solve anything from acne to hip pain. As laughable as that sounds, for some of us it has stopped years of discomfort in its tracks; so, we appreciate your grace as we get over ourselves.

CELIAC DISEASE ENTAILS GOING GLUTEN FREE

For those that are affected by celiac disease, the only truly effective treatment is a 100% gluten-free diet—removing even 99% of gluten from their diet can be insufficient to alleviate all symptoms. Most people who are symptomatic have a reaction from being exposed to less than 50 mg gluten; for perspective, the average Western diet has about 5,000–15,000 mg of gluten per day (Syage et al. 2018, 201).

I have had people say to me, "I thought bread was healthy for you?" I am right there with you—what even happened? Those with asymptomatic celiac disease spend years thinking they are doing right by their bodies while doing just the opposite, to the point that they get diagnosed with celiac disease the usual way, when it is discovered that the villi in their small intestine is flattening to the point of irreversible damage, which can lead to malnutrition and way worse problems than just a distended stomach (which looks oddly similar to a beer gut).

> *Recently, many popular snack foods, beverages, and general products alike are now marketed with the gluten-free label. Trust me, I understand entirely when people think this is just a fad, but for some there is no other option. Gluten is everywhere!*

GLUTEN FREE IS NOT CARB FREE!

Just because a gluten-free food does not contain wheat does not mean that it does not contain carbohydrates. The grains and pseudocereals that are often used in place of wheat, barley, and rye also contain carbohydrates! Food manufacturers typically also add back ample amounts of sugar, milk, and eggs to gluten-free products to make sure they taste great. Gluten-free products are not a miracle cure for weight loss by any stretch of the imagination, but they do at least allow chronic symptoms to subside, and people with celiac disease get to keep their tasty treats and comfort foods. Low-carb or "keto" diets (like the Atkins diet) can work for reasons beyond just cutting back on the sweets and switching your meatball submarine sandwich for a salad. The fact is, most versions of a "healthy diet" now involve much less carbs than they used to—just remember that a gluten-free diet does not necessarily mean a low-carb diet.

That being said, gluten-free grains and pseudocereals like amaranth, buckwheat, millet, quinoa, and teff are showing up in "doctor-recommended diets," and not just for people with gluten intolerance or celiac disease. They contain a wealth of macro- and

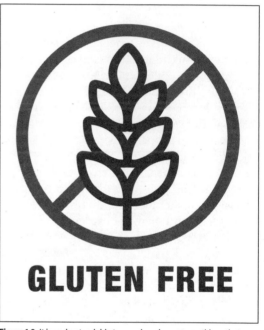

Figure 1.2. It is understandable to wonder why so many things that are naturally gluten free are getting the gluten-free label. This seems to be more of a precaution, but for those who are worried about cross-contamination the label lets them known that the product did not interact with gluten or gluten-containing substances when processed. © Getty/chokkicx

micronutrients and are a great source of protein and fiber (Niro et al. 2019). As any dietitian will tell you, not all calories are created equal. We can say this for carbohydrates too. This is especially true for people with celiac disease or NCGS—a bowl of rice or quinoa and they are just fine, but the moment that person eats farro or couscous there are problems . . . a whole mess of problems. It really is like flicking a nasty switch.

GLUTEN-FREE VERSUS "GLUTEN-REDUCED" BREWING

Currently in the US, "gluten free" means using ingredients that never contained, were derived from, or interacted with gluten from start to finish. The Food and Drug Administration (FDA) came out with its final ruling on gluten-free labeling in the US in August 2020:

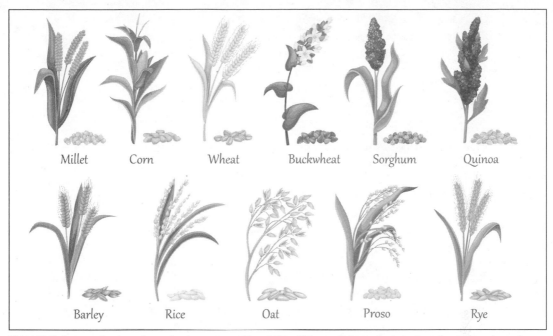

Figure 1.3. Various cereal and pseudocereal grains can be used to make beer. Of these, millet, corn, buckwheat, sorghum, quinoa, rice, and proso (a type of millet) are safe for a person with celiac disease. Wheat, barley, oats, and rye are not safe for someone with celiac disease.
© Getty/setory

> Currently, [the] FDA knows of no scientifically valid analytical method effective in detecting and quantifying with precision the gluten protein content in fermented or hydrolyzed foods in terms of equivalent amounts of intact gluten proteins. Thus, we plan to evaluate compliance of such fermented or hydrolyzed foods that bear a "gluten-free" claim based on records that are made and kept by the manufacturer of the food bearing the "gluten-free" claim and made available to us for inspection and copying. The records need to provide adequate assurance that the food or ingredients used in the food are "gluten-free" before fermentation or hydrolysis. (Food Labeling; Gluten-Free Labeling of Fermented or Hydrolyzed Foods, 85 Fed. Reg. 49,240, 49,241 (Aug. 13, 2020) (amending 21 C.F.R. § 101.91))

Shortly thereafter, in October 2020, the Alcohol and Tobacco Tax and Trade Bureau (TTB) followed with its policy enforcement, TTB Ruling 2020-2, based upon the FDA's final ruling (https://www.ttb.gov/rulings/r2020-2).

ENZYMATIC REDUCTION OF GLUTEN

The 2020 revised ruling of the FDA speaks to the misunderstandings over what makes a product gluten free and how to test such products. This is the case when considering beers that are treated with endopeptidase enzymes, like the one in Brewers Clarex® or Clarity Ferm, which target proline bonds within peptides and proteins. Proline is an amino acid that is particularly frequent in gluten and its derived peptides. Beers with these enzyme products added to them are often marketed as "gluten-reduced." These are typically beers that involve the use of barley, wheat, and rye in the recipe and rely on the added endopeptidases to break down gluten and its derived peptide chains (Lopez and Edens 2005). Endopeptidase enzymes were originally brought to market to reduce chill haze, which occurs when proteins and tannins (polyphenols) come together and become insoluble during cold storage.

The gluten tests vaguely referenced by the FDA and TTB in their labeling guidelines (ELISA R5 Sandwich & Competitive) test for a few specific amino acid sequences, but these enzymes cleave some of the sequences the tests are looking for, creating false negatives and inconclusive results, which we will discuss momentarily.

To the brewing community at large, beers treated with these enzymes appeared promising at first because they appeared to be able to lower gluten levels in beers made with traditional ingredients, namely, barley, wheat, and rye. But subsequent research has shown that the perceived low levels of gluten were due to inadequate testing methods (Tanner et al. 2013; Colgrave et al. 2014). The gluten tests then accepted by the FDA and TTB relied on a procedure called enzyme-linked immunosorbent assay (ELISA). Testing with ELISA relies on antibodies that can detect either whole gluten, prolamins, or prolamin peptide fragments. When testing beers treated with enzymes to reduce gluten, the researchers found that

> ELISA results did not correlate with the relative content of hordein peptides determined by MS [mass spectrometry], **with all barley based beers containing hordein [i.e., gluten]**. We suggest that mass spectrometry is more reliable than ELISA, as ELISA enumerates only the concentration of particular amino-acid epitopes; this may vary between different hordeins and may not be related to the absolute hordein concentration. MS quantification is undertaken using peptides that are specific and unique, enabling the quantification of individual hordein isoforms. This outlines the problem of relying solely on ELISA determination of gluten in beverages such as beer and highlights the need for the development of new sensitive and selective quantitative assay such as MS. (Tanner et al. 2013, 1, under "Conclusions"; emphasis added).

This and other studies, like one conducted by the company that makes Brewers Clarex® (DSM), show that the ELISA test is unreliable even in beers not treated with such an enzyme (Akeroyd et al. 2016, 91).

People with celiac disease and those with gluten intolerance react to certain peptide sequences, regardless of whether the overall gluten protein is intact or not. The study by Colgrave et al. (2014) showed the processing steps that occur in food and beverages containing gluten create a multitude of peptide fragments that can interfere with the detection of those specific fragments that trigger an immune reaction in people with celiac disease. So, while the ELISA cannot necessarily find the important sequences, this does not mean they are not in solution in the final beer and able to affect a person with celiac disease. The group of Colgrave et al. (2014) showed that when a mass spectrometer is used, gluten and reactive gluten peptides could be found in beer samples that had passed the ELISA. This means that a commercial beer that "passed" an ELISA gluten test could contain enough of the problematic peptide sequences to be functionally above the legal limit to be considered gluten free and safe; in some cases, levels detected by mass spectrometry showed these peptides far exceeded the legal limit. (See Appendix A.) The current understanding is that these enzymes do not reduce or remove the offending peptides (Colgrave, Byrne, and Howitt 2017, 9717). These enzymes are really good at reducing beer haze caused by proteins containing large numbers of proline units, which was the original intent. However, products treated with Brewers Clarex® or Clarity Ferm will still start and end with the same amount of gluten peptide sequences. While it may aid in reducing bloating and some of the more acute effects of gluten, people who have celiac disease still have a problem processing these beers, and a certain percentage still react the same (Allred et al. 2017).

What is more, there are currently no clinical trials on "gluten-reduced" beers and their effect on people with problems digesting gluten. One reason for this is that it is difficult to obtain consistent results when testing blood samples from subjects with celiac disease. For example, a 2017 study that looked at the reactivity of celiac patients' sera showed that 6.4% of the study population reacted to barley extract, barley-based beer, and "gluten-reduced" beer, while 12.9% only reacted to the barley and barley-based beer but not necessarily the "gluten-reduced" beer; the control groups showed zero response (Allred et al. 2017, 489–490). While this shows that there are persistent gluten fragments to which some people with celiac disease can react, the findings in that test group from one specific region cannot necessarily be extrapolated to the global population. On top of that, it is possible not every celiac patient in the tested group had antibodies already built up for the test peptide sequences used in the serological study. This means that even without autoimmune symptoms displayed, there could still be damage done if someone with celiac were to consume products made from barley.

PROBLEMS WITH THE "GLUTEN-FREE" LABEL

Regardless of the limitations in assessing the gluten content of commercially produced beer, "gluten-reduced" beers have been around for longer than a decade at this point and are seemingly not going anywhere. Unfortunately, they are marketed directly to people shopping in the gluten-free sections of stores, despite the FDA and TTB explicitly calling them out as *not* gluten free. In fact, any product labeled "gluten-reduced," "crafted to remove gluten," etc., must also include a product safety warning that these products cannot be tested to ensure their safety! The FDA ruling stated:

> Therefore, we have not defined the terms "gluten-reduced," "crafted to remove gluten," or "made to remove gluten," and we do not consider those terms to be equivalent to "gluten-free." (Food Labeling; Gluten-Free Labeling of Fermented or Hydrolyzed Foods, 85 Fed. Reg. 49,240, 49,251 (Aug. 13, 2020))

The TTB in its ruling determined that:

> *Held further,* labels and advertisements may include truthful and accurate statements that the product was "[Processed *or* Treated *or* Crafted] to remove gluten" for products that were fermented from one or more ingredients that are, or are derived from, a gluten-containing grain, where the product is then processed or treated or crafted to remove some or all of the gluten, under the following conditions:
>
> > (1) The following qualifying statement must also appear legibly and conspicuously on the label or in the advertisement as part of (i.e., immediately adjacent to or as a continuation of) the above statement:
> >
> > > "Product fermented from grains containing gluten and [processed *or* treated *or* crafted] to remove gluten. The gluten content of this product cannot be verified, and this product may contain gluten."
>
> (Gluten Content Statements in the Labeling and Advertising of Wine, Distilled Spirits, and Malt Beverages, TTB Ruling 2020-2(V) (Oct. 13, 2020); brackets and italics in the original)

Current TTB rulings never permit the words "gluten-free" to describe a "gluten-reduced" beer. Commercial beer competitions often specify gluten-free categories are for beers meeting TTB's standard for gluten-free. The spirit of TTB's labeling and advertising regulations don't allow mention of a gluten-reduced beer's entry or award in gluten-free categories and doing so could prompt regulatory scrutiny. The bottom line is the TTB regulations aim to keep suppliers from misleading drinkers.

Here are some factors supporting a beer drinker's need for accurate information:
1. The bodily reactions in celiac disease manifest with a huge variety of symptoms (e.g., indigestion, weight gain, hypertension, malnutrition, dermatitis, and depression), so presentation of the disease is multifaceted (Caio et al. 2019, 5–7).

2. When it comes to people with NCGS or celiac disease, symptoms can be different when consuming gluten that has gone through fermentation. Most people I have spoken to directly about this (and my own experience) still manifest gluten-related symptoms when consuming Brewers Clarex-treated barley beer, though these symptoms often differ from the usual reaction caused by ingesting gluten.

3. There is still currently no affordable procedure available that can reliably test for gluten in fermented products. The only reliable method seems to be using a mass spectrometer (Colgrave et al. 2014; Colgrave, Byrne, and Howitt 2017). The lack of precision and corroboration between different ELISA kits accepted by the European Union (EU) to inform "gluten-free" and "low-gluten" labels on products highlights how inadequate testing without the use of mass spectrometry is putting many consumers at risk (Rzychon et al. 2017, 153).

4. There are many people who are wheat intolerant but not barley intolerant, and other permutations of intolerances relating to the barley, wheat, and rye families of grains. This person-to-person variability has confounded scientific understanding and evidence in research (Fasano and Catassi 2001).

Of particular concern is the difference in labeling conventions between the various countries, particularly the large economic zones of the US and the EU and UK. Legislative policy governing labeling should be created for the most vulnerable consumers, hence the final rulings by the FDA and TTB made in 2020 that prohibit a "gluten-reduced" product from being labeled "gluten-free" because current testing methods used by the food and beverage industry cannot accurately quantify the gluten content of such products (85 Fed. Reg. 49,240; TTB Ruling 2020-2). In the EU and UK, however, such products are allowed to be labeled "gluten free" despite them possibly containing levels of gluten much higher than safe thresholds due to inaccuracies and uncertainties inherent in the ELISA testing kits commercially available (Rzychon et al. 2017). Essentially, since ELISA is the best food-grade test available at the moment, these legislative bodies are willing to roll the dice.

These discrepancies between a "gluten-reduced" product that is labeled "gluten-free" and the actual level of gluten that may be present in it is extremely worrying for people with celiac disease who are trying to manage their condition. To compound the issue, some people with celiac disease do not react acutely to gluten-reduced beers, which makes many people believe that these products are safe. Since it is a progressive disease, a person with celiac disease may be able to tolerate these beers initially while still causing irreparable damage to their small intestine.[2]

When producers are allowed to label a product that is known to contain gluten as "gluten-free," it could potentially be doing more damage than necessary to the consumer. The best way to think about this is to consider another serious food allergy: peanut allergy. You would not walk up to someone with an allergy like that and offer them a product labeled "peanut-reduced," let alone try to pass them off as "peanut-free" . . . would you?

In light of the lack of a reliable gluten test used by the food and beverage industry, you could be forgiven for wondering about the ethics of "gluten-reduced" beers being called gluten-free. "Gluten-reduced" or "crafted to remove gluten" are, in my opinion, misleading statements at best, though legally allowed. At any rate, people who are consuming these products are essentially participating in an international experiment, since research is stacking up to show that the enzymatic removal of gluten is ineffective and the standard industry testing methods to ensure it has been effective do not work. People with celiac disease that drink these beverages are risking their own health, plain and simple. Such products are unsafe for all people with celiac disease or gluten intolerance to consume.[3]

[2] Lori Welstead, "Gluten Removed/Reduced Beer: Safety Concerns for Those with Celiac Disease," Dietitian's Corner, *Impact*, October 2016, https://www.cureceliacdisease.org/wp-content/uploads/CdC_Newsletter_2016_Issue03_FINAL-1.pdf.

[3] Sam Lemonick, "A New Test to Make Sure Your Beer Is Gluten Free," *Forbes*, Nov 1, 2017, 2:58 a.m. EDT, https://www.forbes.com/sites/samlemonick/2017/11/01/a-new-test-to-make-sure-your-beer-is-gluten-free/.

Truly, the only effective method when it comes to removing gluten from our beer is to produce it from 100% gluten-free ingredients. It is understandable that brewers have sought to find a simple and inexpensive process that would render their beers safe for more consumers; however, much as alchemists found in their search for the philosopher's stone that easily turns lead into gold, such a process does not seem to exist.

TRULY GLUTEN-FREE BREWING
Did somebody say not all carbs are created equal? From a brewing standpoint, the high incidence of carbohydrates in gluten-free grains makes them ideal for brewing.

CONSIDERATIONS WHEN USING GLUTEN-FREE GRAINS
Certain intrinsic characteristics of gluten-free grains have nuances that affect their use in beer recipes:
1. A much smaller grain size. This can change lautering considerations, as most false bottoms are calibrated to the larger, huskier barley grain. While grains slipping through is an issue, a bigger challenge can be wort channeling and grain bed collapse.
2. Many pseudocereals have a high β-glucan (beta-glucan) content, specifically quinoa and buckwheat, which can create stuck mashes if not treated properly.
3. Many of these ingredients are not even grains at all! This includes lentils, sunflower seeds, and sweet potatoes, for instance.
4. A much lower enzymatic content. This is an important point, which we will get into at length. Many have complained that you need to be a chemistry wiz or something just to brew this way. It is true that many pioneers in this space, in fact, are such wizzes; however, things have changed drastically based on new brewing tactics, the availability of malts and other ingredients, as well as increased availability of enzymes and proteases that can be added.
5. With the variety of gluten-free grains, pseudocereals, and other fermentable adjuncts used, there are necessarily different mash methods that may be used. This means there is not (nor can there be) a consensus on any specific mash method among the gluten-free brewing community.

ENSURING YOU BREW GLUTEN FREE
It is not that hard to start brewing gluten-free beers, as long as the ingredients you use are from trusted suppliers that do not share specific equipment with gluten-containing ingredients. For example, if a mill is used on barley grains, any naturally gluten-free grains passed through that same mill can be rendered unsafe due to cross contamination. Depending on the supplier and how the grains were treated, ingredients that normally would be considered safe—specifically, flaked rice, corn, and some oats—might not be that safe when buying from a general brewing supplier or your local homebrew store. Non-porous surfaces like stainless steel and some others are safe if properly cleaned in between use. As with most of the know-how in gluten-free brewing, the real treasure troves when sourcing ingredients are found outside of the usual channels.

If you have already brewed barley-based beer on your existing system, there are some additional considerations. To start, a best practice is to dedicate a set of soft materials in your brewhouse to gluten-free brewing. This includes hoses, gaskets, and basically anything else that is not metal. Some breweries have even gone as far as dedicating a whole separate space in the brewery to gluten-free brewing, specifically where barley dust is a cross-contamination risk. Depending on the design, false bottoms are also worth changing out, as barley can often be found hidden in crevices. In any case, the average false bottom slits are too wide for gluten-free malts and grains.

DEDICATED GLUTEN-FREE VERSUS 100% GLUTEN-FREE
Dedicated gluten-free breweries are those that only produce gluten-free products on dedicated gluten-free equipment. That means no gluten or ingredients containing gluten are allowed in the facility.

At time of writing, there were 21 breweries in North America producing gluten-free beer in a dedicated facility (table 1.2).

Table 1.2. The 100% Dedicated Gluten Free Breweries

Alt Brew	Madison, Wisconsin
Aurochs Brewing Co.	Emsworth, Pennsylvania
Beliveau Farm	Blacksburg, Virginia
Bierly Brewing	McMinnville, Oregon
Brewery Nyx	Grand Rapids, Michigan
Buck Wild Brewing	Oakland, California
Burning Brothers Brewing	St. Paul, Minnesota
Dark Hills Brewing Company	Seligman, Missouri
Divine Science Brewing	Tustin, California
Dos Luces Brewery	Denver, Colorado
Eckert Malting & Brewing	Chico, California
Evasion Brewing	McMinnville, Oregon
Ghostfish Brewing Company	Seattle, Washington
Ground Breaker Brewing	Portland, Oregon
Holidaily Brewing Company	Golden, Colorado
Lucky Pigeon Brewing Co.	Biddeford, Maine
Moonshrimp Brewing	Portland, Oregon
Mutantis Brewery	Portland, Oregon
NEFF Brewing	Tulsa, Oklahoma
Red Leaf Gluten-Free Brewing	Jeffersonville, Vermont
Rolling Mill Brewery	Middleton, Ohio

Source: BestGlutenFreeBeers.com

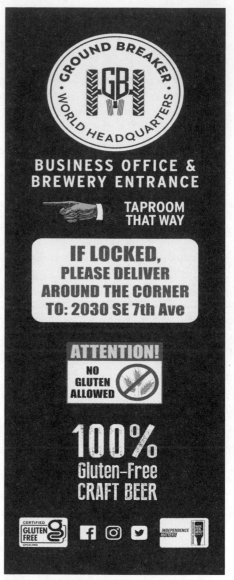

Figure 1.4. Dedicated gluten-free facilities, like Ground Breaker Brewing in Portland, OR, even have signs on the outside of their building to state it. *Courtesy of Ground Breaker Brewing & Gastropub*

If you are a commercial brewer, you can legally make 100% gluten-free beer in a barley-based brewery, but the cleaning standards need to be beyond the regulatory minimum standards (MBAA 2018), and the grain should be bought pre-milled from a certified supplier unless you have a separate mill and auger for gluten-free grains exclusively. This is so that you can keep a record that the product was tested before hydrolysis or fermentation and shown to be at the right level. Taking these precautions helps better ensure compliance with FDA regulations by minimizing possible areas where cross contamination can occur, and often shows that steps beyond the regulatory minimum standards were taken in good faith. Some barley breweries have incorporated smaller, separate pilot systems specifically for brewing 100% gluten-free beers. However, dedicated gluten-free breweries hold themselves to the higher standard of dedicated equipment in a dedicated space to fully remove the risk of cross contamination.

> *If you are looking to make "gluten-reduced" beer, even after the warnings above, there are a ton of Brewer's Publications books that feature incredible recipes from accomplished barley brewers. Use any barley-based recipe and add Brewers Clarex® or Clarity Ferm. However, please understand the risks associated with this style of brewing. Off-the-shelf gluten testing kits are not reliable in fermented or hydrolyzed products like beer, kombucha, or pickles. They are, however, reliable when used on ingredients pre-fermentation, if you want to see just how much gluten truly is in a barley-based beer.*

Through this book, I will show you how fun and rewarding gluten-free brewing is, in part because it takes many of "sacred" rules from conventional grain brewing and smashes them to bits! We will be exploring the various ingredients available to gluten-free brewers, various recipe considerations, as well as taking a deep dive into the plethora of available grains. *There are more types of grain that do not contain gluten than ones that do!*

Fasten your seatbelt, as you are about to expand your brewing repertoire, your palate, and your understanding of gluten-free ingredients, their history, and true place in brewing.

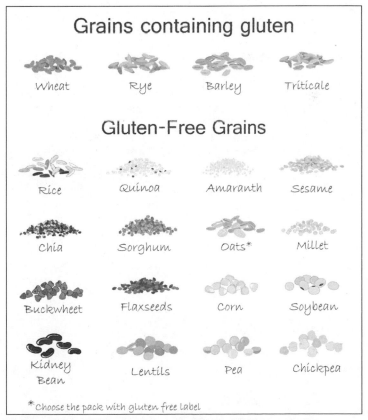

Figure 1.5. The types of gluten-free grains easily outnumber those that contain gluten.
*Note: approximately 20% of people with celiac disease have been found to react to oats.
© Getty/Toltemara

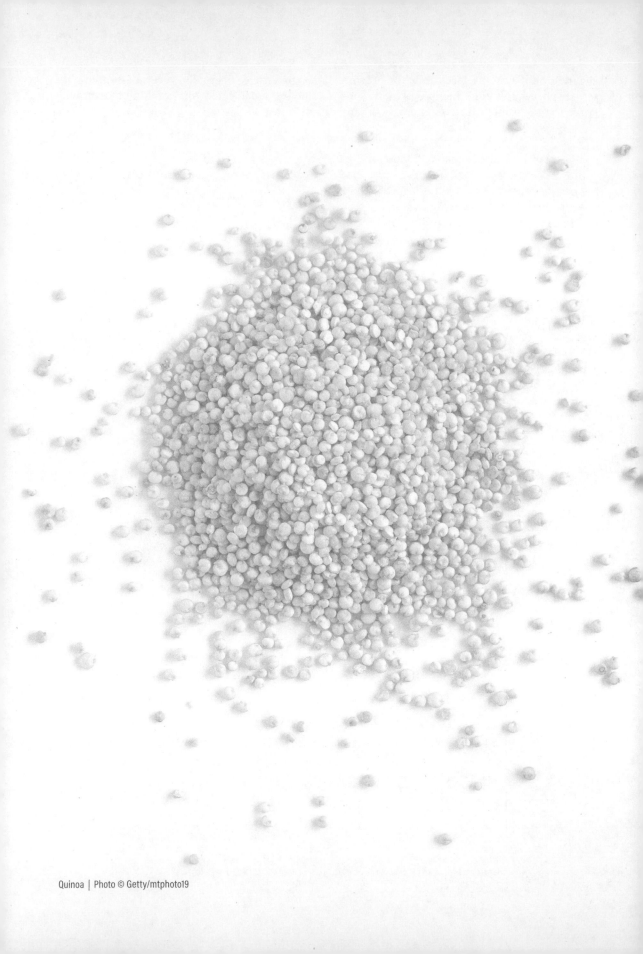

Quinoa | Photo © Getty/mtphoto19

Available Ingredients: An Overview

SOURCING INGREDIENTS

Luckily for brewers of gluten-free beers, there are technically more types of grains (if you count pseudocereals) that do not contain gluten than grains that do contain gluten. The question becomes, which ingredients are the right ones to choose when you just really miss *beer*? I contend that humans have always had the ability to use any ingredient to create beer, whether with sorghum and millet in Africa, corn and quinoa in South America, or pineapple and agave in Central America. You also have the law on your side to defend that. In a 2008 ruling, the US Alcohol and Tobacco Tax and Trade Bureau (TTB) stated:

> Section 5052(a) of the IRC (26 U.S.C. 5052(a)) defines the term "beer," for purposes of Chapter 51, as "beer, ale, porter, stout, and other similar fermented beverages (including saké or similar products) of any name or description containing one-half of 1 percent or more of alcohol by volume, brewed or produced from malt, wholly or in part, or from any substitute therefor." Essentially the same definition appears in the TTB regulations at 27 CFR 25.11. In addition, with reference to what may be a substitute for malt, § 25.15(a) of the TTB regulations (27 CFR 25.15(a)) states that "[o]nly rice, grain of any kind, bran, glucose, sugar, and molasses are substitutes for malt." (Classification of Brewed Products, TTB Ruling 2008-3, p. 3, July 7, 2008)

"Grain of any kind" is a workable substitute, and therefore the many gluten-free grains available are allowed to be in any home or professional brewer's arsenal. But for those who are familiar with craft beer and its taste, the conversation will undoubtedly lead to a pivotal question: *What substitute is an exact replacement for barley?* Sure, we can call it a *substitute*, but most people expect *replacement*. Just because it is legally beer does not mean it has world class potential.

As a novice brewer of gluten-free beer, I learned quickly I would not be able to just make gluten-free beer taste like the craft beer I was used to, at least not overnight . . . As such, I thought the best way to start this chapter is to discuss my first foray in gluten-free brewing. My initial grain bill, which was for a five-gallon recipe, consisted of the following:

- 5.0 lb. rolled oats*
- 1.0 lb. sorghum syrup
- 1.0 lb. honey
- 1.0 lb. brown rice syrup
- 0.5 lb. flaked corn (which accidentally got added during the boil)

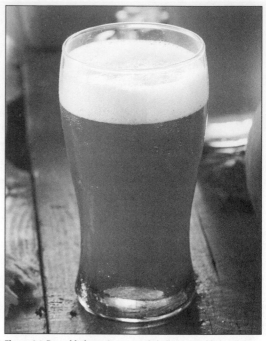

Figure 2.1. Pumpkin beer. Some people believe pumpkin beer was served at the first Thanksgiving. They theorize that pumpkin was used because the barley crop had not yet ripened. © *Getty/bhofack2*

* Making sure the oats are certified gluten-free is a big deal, as cross contamination is so hard to avoid that the oats have to be grown in a field that has never grown wheat before. But even still, the avenin in oats can still activate the same immune response as does barley in a significant minority of people with celiac disease (Hardy et al. 2015, 59–60).

This was supposed to be an easy drinking blonde ale between 3.6% and 4.2% ABV. Knowing what I know today, the grain bill was a commendably brave attempt for a first-time gluten-free beer brewer! This is due to the special treatment required for so many unmalted oats in a recipe of that size, particularly the enzymes you would need: proteases for mash drainage (rice hulls would of course be essential, even with exogenous enzymes, since rolled oats do not have a husk) and amylases for extracting any sugar from the oats. If you are a beginner, I definitely recommend using extracts for this recipe and wait until you have a few successful fermentations under your belt before you go adding that many rolled oats.

The truth about this beer was that, due to mistakes in the brewing process, all I was able to do was create an unfermentable sludge pile. This was down to the added flaked corn combining with the oat slurry that was created in the boil from improper lautering. For some reason, it also had an ominously gray color . . . In all honesty, I should have done a lot more homework before getting started. The funny part for me was that I was borrowing a friend's homebrew system, and he had brewed before—we just did not know the right thing to do without barley at the time. He helped me figure things out from there.

The good news is, you do not have to be like me! There are websites like Gluten Free Home Brewing (https://www.glutenfreehomebrewing.com) and Gluten Free Brew Supply (https://gfbsupply.com) that have been around for some time now. Their selection of ingredients is also incredible! There are so many different flavors and varieties that you might not know what to do at first. But never fear—on top of the ingredients, these websites carry articles and videos, and they can provide quality instructions even if you do not buy a kit. From malts, to hops, to syrups, adjuncts, and yeast, everything they sell is gluten free. This magic, however, does come with a price, especially for those living outside of North America. For some, the cost can be prohibitive. Although suppliers like Gluten Free Home Brewing may offer bulk pricing, base malts still cost around $3.33/lb. without shipping—I know for many, that is a tough monetary pill to swallow.

The goal of this chapter is to make sure you can make great beer, no matter where you are. Regardless of which country you find yourself in, there are gluten-free ingredients for sale, and you can always cultivate and malt your own. For example, if you live in a tropical climate then you might have easy access to grains like corn, amaranth, and rice; perhaps these are even more readily available than barley, and you may also have easy access to fruits and purees. Local sourcing is everything in brewing! Where hops are hard to come by, tea leaves, spices, orange peels, etc. can serve a similar purpose in your beers. Even if this is your first time, you have a long line of brewers who came before you who used such ingredients.

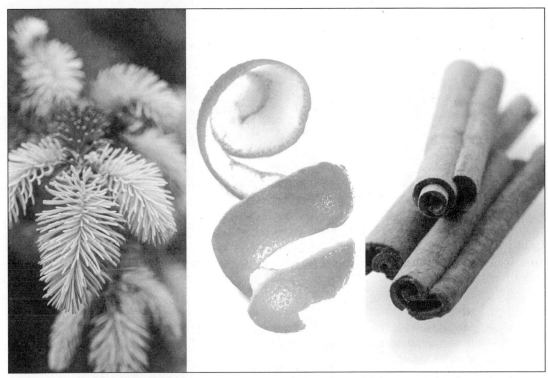

Figure 2.2. Spruce tips, orange peel, cinnamon. Many ingredients like spruce tips, orange peel, and cinnamon have been flavoring beer for a lot longer than hops have. © *Getty/Oksana_Schmidt (spruce); Getty/designsstock (orange); Getty/Alexandra Draghici (cinnamon)*

In the US, Europe, and Australia/New Zealand, selecting ingredients from your local homebrew store might be more confusing, potentially even dangerous, because of cross contamination. Although some of the ingredients you will find did start off as gluten free, they may not be when you buy them. Trustworthy producers will typically get certification as well as dedicate equipment and processing facilities to gluten-free grains. It is worth doing your research if you react adversely to gluten. Producers often are not aware of cross contamination concerns, and it may take pointing this out to them to bring about an update to their practices. Still an amazing resource if you have one, here is a list of what I would say is probably safe at just about any local homebrew store, *if the ingredient is still sealed in its original packaging*:

Rice hulls. Rice hulls are great for drainage, and for beginners they can be a great consideration or failsafe when performing a lauter or sparge with some ingredients. Although rice hulls are unfermentable, they can help bring peace of mind to brewers who are worried about stuck mashes. Assuming they are gluten-free, they are likely one of the only safe grain elements that you can buy at a homebrew store.

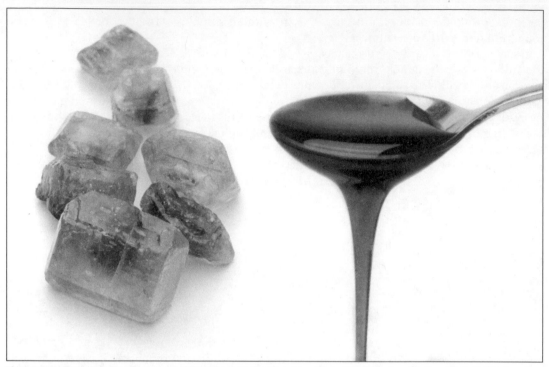

Figure 2.3. Candi sugars and syrups are good additions for gluten-free beers to provide body and extra fermentables. © *Getty/Natikka (sugar); Getty/illusionsteam (syrup)*

Candi sugar/syrup. Candi sugar and syrup are good for adding color, as well as certain aromas and flavors. They are highly recommended for the beginner brewer, as they can help boost ABV when you are still figuring out your best method for extracting fermentables from gluten-free grains.

Rice syrup solids. Rice syrup solids are another great tool for adding fermentable material without affecting the flavor. But beware—the lack of flavor means you will need to figure out some other source of character flavors.

Sorghum syrup. I have seen sorghum syrup available in some stores, although certainly not all, so I would not rely on this—but when you see it, buy it. The sorghum syrup you will see is typically supplied by Briess, and they make it from white sorghum. This Briess product is made from unmalted grains but touted as having a high maltose and free amino nitrogen (FAN) content. The FAN content is still two-thirds that of regular malt, and you will need to consider adding FAN-containing yeast nutrient when using this syrup.

> *These three fermentables—candi sugar, rice syrup solids, and sorghum syrup—are great to have on hand in case you run into any problems, say, with an all-grain mash that does not go according to plan.*

Hops. As a gluten-free homebrewer who is worried about cross contamination, hops are one of the only reasons I go to the local homebrew store. Hops are naturally gluten free, and hop growers rarely process malt as well. Make sure the hops you buy have not been repackaged in the shop, where grain dust is pervasive!

Maltodextrin. Maltodextrin, in both its corn and tapioca-based forms, is great for adding body and residual sweetness to gluten-free beers. Using maltodextrin helps you get close to certain styles because it can add "chewiness" and "stickiness" to the end product. In addition, dextrins help promote head retention in gluten-free beers. **However**, maltodextrin is often made from wheat, even though it can be marketed as gluten-free due to the method of processing used. Some consumers do not consider it a safe product, despite it being labeled gluten free.

Lactose. Lactose is another great adjunct for adding body and creaminess, and it is something unfermentable in the wort that can help lend additional sweetness to the resulting beer. Akin to maltodextrin, lactose will help your beer be thicker and likely contribute to head retention. Note that many people who are gluten intolerant are also allergic to dairy and may have a reaction to lactose.

Yeast. In general, dry yeasts are produced gluten free and are labeled as such, including some (not all) those made by Fermentis, Lallemand, Danstar, Mangrove Jack's, and Gozdawa. Liquid yeast brands, like those from Wyeast and White Labs, are propagated in media containing barley (barley maltodextrin, typically). There are some brands, such as Propagate Labs in Colorado, that have begun offering their liquid yeast strains raised on gluten-free media using dedicated equipment to gluten-free producers if requested, but there may still be limited yeasts available due to limited supply, distribution, or available strains. Gluten Free Home Brewing does group buys of gluten-free liquid yeasts when available—make sure to participate in their annual surveys so that you get the yeast you are looking for.

Yeast nutrient. Tread lightly and research each brand before you buy, but yeast nutrient is a good way to make sure you have a great tasting beer no matter what ingredient you use: "Happy fermentation, happy beer," as the saying goes. The concern with yeast nutrient is that spent yeast previously propagated on barley medium can often find its way into a nutrient mixture. Many packages might not list ingredients, so you will need to go to the brand's web page to check. Additionally, many drinkers who are gluten

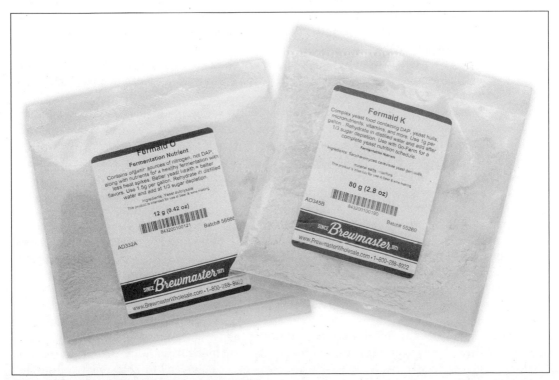

Figure 2.4. These two types of yeast nutrients are known to be safe.

intolerant are also allergic or react to soy and dairy—several common yeast nutrients have both.

Brewing salts. Naturally gluten free like hops, water salts are another great reason to shop at the local homebrew store. Various ingredients will affect the taste of your beer downstream, including brewing salts. For example, adding calcium chloride to a soft water profile will emphasize the maltiness of your beer. Conversely, adding calcium sulfate will emphasize crispness and hop-derived flavors, including bitterness.

Miscellaneous. Additional ingredients like spices and purees are also naturally gluten free, but these can also be purchased from other places as well.

Bottling, fermenting, brewing, and other packaging supplies are of course a great resource and why the LHBS is necessary, but you will likely need to search elsewhere to get all the ingredients you need for brewing gluten-free beer.

WHICH GRAINS MAKE IT BEER ANYWAY?

We've answered some basic questions, but still haven't even touched, "What grain can I buy that is a substitute for barley?"

Throughout the gluten-free brewing world, homebrew and commercial, there is currently no consensus on a standard base beer recipe. Homebrewers in Africa and Australia often use different grain bills from people in North America and Europe, for example. Commercially available gluten-free beers in different parts of the US are another great example: Ground Breaker Brewing in Portland, OR has its signature blend of lentils, chestnuts, and sorghum; Aurochs Brewing in Pittsburgh, PA blends millet and quinoa; and Dos Luces in Denver, CO pays homage to ancient chicha (corn beer) and pulque (agave beer made from maguey) in their modern brews. These are all drastically different interpretations of gluten-free beer.

From the perspective of judging beer in competitions, wrangling these disparate beers into a single style category creates its own challenges. A judge at the gluten-free category table could easily taste eight different lagers brewed with eight different grain bases. At that point, what is and what is not an off-flavor? If it is not barley-based does that just automatically mean it has an *off*-flavor? Possibly so—yet commercial brewers have been able to produce beers that cleanly create the flavors of traditional beers, including lagers. Take, for example, a "wheat beer" that is brewed gluten free without wheat: as someone who used to go crazy for all wheat-based styles before having to give up gluten, this is one of the easiest styles to consistently recreate gluten free as a homebrewer.

However, despite the above, certain fermentables will always provide unique flavors not found in barley malt. Given that some of these flavors aren't really recognized in many style categories, this puts brewing with certain gluten-free grains into uncharted territory at times. The world is your oyster in this brave new world of gluten-free brewing, from cereals and pseudocereals to things that are not grain: nuts like chestnuts, seeds like sunflower seeds, legumes like soybeans and lentils, and root vegetables like sweet potatoes. As you can imagine, these will all elicit completely different tastes from barley, wheat, or rye, and that can be a good thing!

This may be an obvious statement, but no matter what the ingredient is, you will of course not be using barley or wheat when brewing gluten free. With the variety in tastes available, I believe it may be possible to transcend classic styles altogether, to the point that some traditional beer names may be insufficient. All that being said, there are some good like-for-like gluten-free beer substitutions to be found.

The assumption that beers require barley malt is clearly myopic, and forgets the rich history that beer brings to the table. The popularity of lager and ale styles that originated from Europe is largely due to the extent of European colonization and industrialization over the preceding three or four centuries. Many natively European beers that were made from things like fruit, tree sap, and vegetables are nearly extinct themselves. Nearly every colonized or subsumed culture had developed their own defined styles of beer prior to the arrival of popular European styles, and they were often 100% gluten free! These styles exhibited their own rich and specialized flavors. Though these ingredients featured more prominently in brewing in an era since long gone, when blended with modern flavors and techniques they can both achieve style profiles typically associated with barley and present opportunities for new (or reimagined) styles to come in the future. Maybe the current barley-based standard is a glass ceiling worth shattering . . .

> *Styles with yeast-dominated flavors are typically easier to recreate gluten free. But certain gluten-free grains can also contribute elements complimentary to styles normally considered to have "clean" fermentation profiles; for example, corn, tapioca, and rice syrup solids have been featured in adjunct lagers for quite some time.*

COMMONLY AVAILABLE INGREDIENTS

With respect to the varied palette of ingredients that follows, I will say that six base grains dominate the many domestic and international gluten-free beers on the market today. The six are sorghum, rice, millet, corn, buckwheat, and quinoa, although buckwheat and quinoa will typically feature as less than 30% of the grist. These ingredients, when used effectively, have been shown capable of creating beers that are nearly indistinguishable from their gluten-containing counterparts.

Many of the malts discussed in this chapter are from specialist US malthouses, many of whom ship internationally. What is even better is that new malthouses have sprung up in other territories, including Ovunque in Argentina and The AltGrain Co. in the UK.

Wherever you are, tap into your local agricultural community. If there are certain ingredients that are easier to source, they might be worth becoming your base ingredient. Then spend the real money on specialty malts from a dedicated malthouse (unless you can malt it and roast it at home yourself).

CEREAL GRAINS

Sorghum (extract, raw, and malted forms). By most accounts (my own experience included), sorghum has a quasi-malty-bitter taste. It can have a distinct flavor in beer, often described imprecisely as "sorghum twang." Sorghum has been used for thousands of years in Africa as a brewing grain, most commonly without hops and soured. It is also used to make *baijiu*, a spirit commonly consumed in China, thus making it the most widely consumed spirit in the world.[1] Its malty bitterness gives sorghum beers exceptional flavor and drinkability when brewed both traditionally and with a modern take. Sorghum grows well in both its motherland of Africa as well as China and the US.

Since many of the first gluten-free beers in the US market featured sorghum, its unique flavor

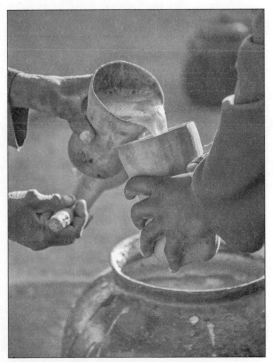

Figure 2.5. African Sorghum Beer, known by many names, is typically opaque in appearance. It can often be as thick and viscous as porridge, as many traditional recipes do not separate the grain from the wort before fermentation. © *Getty/poco_bw*

---

[1] Julie Wernau, "World's Most Consumed Liquor Tries to Make It in the U.S.," *Wall Street Journal*, Oct. 14, 2018, 11:00 a.m. ET, https://www.wsj.com/articles/worlds-most-consumed-liquor-tries-to-make-it-in-the-u-s-1539529200 [subscription required].

dominates most people's understanding of how gluten-free grains taste. In the US, sorghum is easiest to source in its syrup/extract form, but that is starting to change as some malthouses are beginning to offer sorghum malt. It is commonly used as a base malt, with an extract potential of 33 gravity points per pound per gallon (PPG) malted and 35 PPG as a syrup (equivalent to 275 and 292 l°/kg, respectively). Its malted form appears to have the cleanest flavor profile.

Certain people remark that they can pick up a green apple or metallic taste from sorghum syrup-based beers, which can be exacerbated by poor yeast health. One of the biggest considerations when using sorghum extract is the low level of FAN relative to barley malt. You may want to add additional grains other than sorghum to the grain bill or add an appropriate yeast nutrient to maintain yeast health during fermentation. If gluten-free yeast nutrients are hard to come by, oxygenating your wort prior to fermentation will at least give your yeast the best chance to ferment your beer cleanly without the off-flavors that can occur.

Whether brewing traditional, modern, or indigenous styles of beer, I would advise leaning into the natural flavors sorghum elicits. Sorghum is praised for its sustainability, as it can grow in soils in which barley has trouble.

Rice. Rice is available raw or malted and kilned to varying degrees. It can be found in most grocery stores, but grocery store-bought rice will need special treatment. Many stores will carry it in extract form as brown rice syrup. Malted rice has a great beer-like neutral grain taste in its pale form, and there are crystal and roast rice malts that provide great color and character for many beer styles. It is, pound for pound, a reliable base malt in gluten-free brewing, with an extract potential of 31 PPG (259 l°/kg).

Some people have detected spicy, earthy, and even wintergreen or celery-like aromas and tastes in their finished rice beers. The first half of that list sounds pretty good, but wintergreen and celery? These two flavors appear to arise because rice often lacks enough protein and FAN for the yeast to be able to complete fermentation (somewhat similar to sorghum). Personally, I have had to re-pitch yeast on some all-rice beers to make sure they have fermented all the way out. I would advise using a yeast nutrient, as well as

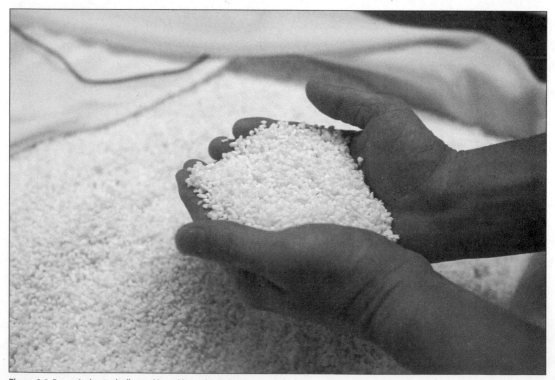

Figure 2.6. Brewer's rice, typically used in making sake. © *Getty/gyro*

including another grain or pseudocereal with a higher protein content to ensure you achieve the desired beer-like qualities you are looking for, such as clean grain tastes and lasting head retention, especially if you do not have access to enzymes that can pull components other than sugar from the rice.

When unmalted, rice grains can really mess with your expected mash efficiencies if you do not burst the endosperm. White sushi rice is even worse from a sparge standpoint. Many gluten-free brewers have seen an increase in efficiency by utilizing enzymes that incorporate a pullulanase (described further in chapter 5). These enzymes can gelatinize the starches in rice, which removes the need for a cereal mash, and pulls head-stabilizing compounds and FAN-promoting precursors into solution.

Rice needs a longer mash time with special enzymes; even then, a higher resting temperature will aid in liquefaction and gelatinization, and set you up properly for starch solubilization and degradation. Starch degradation into soluble and fermentable sugars is what makes beer.

Rice benefits from a cocktail of enzymes like pullulanase, lipase, cellulase, and amylase. The development of these enzyme products has allowed rice to become an even more promising grain for brewing. When I first started out brewing, rice had a lower extract potential than millet and buckwheat, and now it has more!

> I have been able to make a delicious and complex 12% ABV all-grain, all-rice malt beer with notes of vanilla and smoke (along with an interesting clove taste, which I typically associate more with buckwheat).

Millet. Millet is available raw or malted and kilned, with various crystal and specialty roast versions sold. From a brewing standpoint, you will typically only find the white or red varieties of proso millet (*Panicum miliaceum*). Although there are many other species of millet which you can (in theory) use for brewing, they might not be as reliable a base malt as proso millet. In the US, white proso millet is the easiest to find and comes in at least 20 types of malt. These malts provide flavors ranging from malty and sweet (bready, biscuity, caramel) to dark and roasted (chocolate, coffee), which will be discussed further in chapter 3.

Proso millet has been selectively targeted in the last 10 years as a great potential gluten-free malt, specifically because it has relatively high levels of α-amylase (alpha-amylase) when compared with other gluten-free grains. However, given a diastatic power of 40 degrees Lintner—compared to 80–120°Lintner for most barley base malts—and higher gelatinization temperature, mashing millet without the use of additional enzymes can leave unfermentable sugars remaining in the beer. (Diastatic power refers to the enzymatic power of the malt, that is, the malt's ability to break down starches into simpler fermentable sugars during the mashing process.)

Many brewers just ignore millet's own (endogenous) enzymes entirely and rely instead on added (exogenous) enzymes. To get the full extract potential from a grain like millet, the

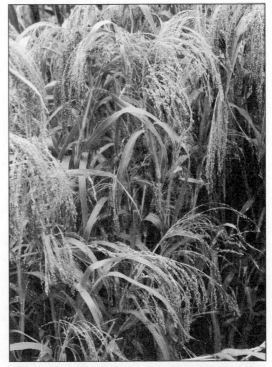

Figure 2.7. Proso millet, the most commonly available brewing millet in North America. © *Getty/enjoynz*

"magic" mash temperature rest does seem to be 170–175°F (76–79°C) due to the high gelatinization temperature of the starch. That is why an exogenous high-temperature α-amylase is often used, as the endogenous α-amylases denature at this temperature. Hence, when brewing with millet it is recommended to use at least two types of enzymes (or a cocktail of enzymes) in concert with the grain's endogenous enzymes to make sure the beer ferments well and to its expected finishing gravity. You will likely need to use a rising temperature step mash or falling temperature step mash (discussed in chapter 5) with millet to get the most out of the endogenous and exogenous enzymes, because most enzymes work best below 160°F (71°C).

Like barley, wheat, and rye, millet has a fairly high friability. This makes malted millet a reliable base malt in gluten-free brewing, because its endosperm can be fully crushed in milling (as opposed to grains like rice that still need a cereal mash or pullulanase-containing enzymes to extract the necessary soluble starches). In fact, millet is so friable it can get a little bit powdery at times, so using rice hulls or a custom screen on the mash is often advised by producers. If using rice hulls, up to about 1 lb. for every 7 lb. of grain seems to make the most sense. When brewing at the commercial scale, I like to call the first 10 minutes of vorlauf (wort recirculation) the "milky time." If left unhydrolyzed, this suspended grain powder can create a film or sludge on the top of your mash bed, which can cause wort channeling that lowers your extract efficiency (because less of the sugary goodness is separated from your grain) or—worse—a stuck mash.

Corn (maize). Corn, or maize (*Zea mays*), as it is grown today has a couple of varieties typically meant for human consumption that come in a diverse range of colors. These varieties are available for brewing in both raw and malted forms, with some roast malts now available.

Yellow corn. Yellow corn has a wonderfully sweet, slight creamy note when raw and flaked, but malted yellow corn can also have a crisp, clean, and malty taste. Corn's true extract potential is disputed and seems to depend on the techniques employed: some resources say 39 PPG (325 l°/kg) for flaked corn (Palmer 2017, 289) but malted corn will be less. Grouse Malt House has been able to achieve 27 PPG (225 l°/kg) using a fairly simple falling temperature mash and exogenous enzymes (chapter 5). I say if you treat malted or unmalted yellow corn right you can reliably get about 29 PPG (242 l°/kg). This treatment involves milling it with one or two passes and cooking it—either literally cooking it during the mash by incorporating a cereal adjunct mash step, or by using exogenous enzymes that lower the gelatinization temperature. Properly handled, yellow corn can make the final product just sing when you taste it.

Blue corn and red corn. Blue corn and red corn elicit more of an earthy or herbal, stone fruit-like taste (from what I have tasted) in addition to the traditional corn sweetness. Whatever the case, the color can often play tricks on the palate, as these colors scream "grape" and "cherry" in the brain. In my experience using it as a base malt in chicha, I'd say you can reliably get 22 PPG (184 l°/kg) from Grouse Malt House's malted blue corn. Malted blue corn goes well with any "barnyard" yeasts (e.g., *Brettanomyces* or *Pichia* species), saison yeasts, or Belgian/phenolic ale yeasts. The rich fruity and spicy flavors and aromas that these yeasts put off in conjunction with blue corn make for some of the most unique beers I have ever tasted. Yeast strains of the genus *Pichia* are used in traditionally fermented chicha.

Oats. Oats can be found in raw, rolled, steel cut, malted, and, now, certified gluten-free malted versions, with some roasts and caramels/crystals coming to market. Malted oats are known for bringing a sharp, biscuity or malty taste, while raw or rolled oats have a creamy texture. Raw oats typically never get used in sufficient quantities in a grist to care about extract, but malted oats can contribute at least 25 PPG (209 l°/kg) to your grain bill.

You should reach out to any supplier of oat malt to make sure the oats are certified gluten free, as they are often processed on shared farm and malthouse equipment. I am aware that many in the gluten-free community believe oats do not belong in gluten-free beer because the gliadin-like protein found in oats, avenin, causes adverse effects in many people with celiac disease (see chapter 1). This is 100% understandable, and if oats are not on the menu for you, do not worry about it.

For those like me that can handle oats, it is a grain that almost guarantees lacing on your beer glass when used in its malted form due to its high protein content. Although oats do have a high β-glucan (beta-glucan) content as well, that does not necessarily guarantee a cloudy beer (consider that barley has one of the highest levels of β-glucan and still makes clear beer). Just like with any other grain, performing a protein rest and a vorlauf can help clear an oat beer. Another great thing is that oats have a kernel size similar to rice, so they are great for improving the drainage of any mash. When used as a base malt, oats can contribute a honey-like flavor profile in the end beer.

Teff. Not commonly used outside of Africa, most anecdotal accounts of teff talk about it being more trouble than it's worth, although recent research suggests levels of β-amylase (beta-amylase) are high enough in teff that it could be a viable grain for brewing with the correct mashing technique (Ledley et al. 2021). This is one grain that I do not have much experience with, though that shouldn't dissuade you from trying it out. Similar to quinoa, because of the kernel's small stature, teff may be best suited to puffing in a skillet before mashing.

PSEUDOCEREALS

Quinoa. Quinoa has always been easy to find in raw form at the grocery or health food store, but now it is available flaked as well. Quinoa is a seed that is prepared like a grain, although botanically speaking it is more closely related to chard or spinach. In its flaked form, quinoa is great for any grain bill, providing 31 PPG (259 l°/kg). The seeds are small and do not have much husk, so you may want to consider puffing quinoa on your skillet before mashing with it at home, if you are only able to find it at the store.

Quinoa contributes a peppery, spicy flavor, though it can turn vegetal at times. As with many pseudocereals, quinoa is great for adding body and head retention due to its high levels of protein,

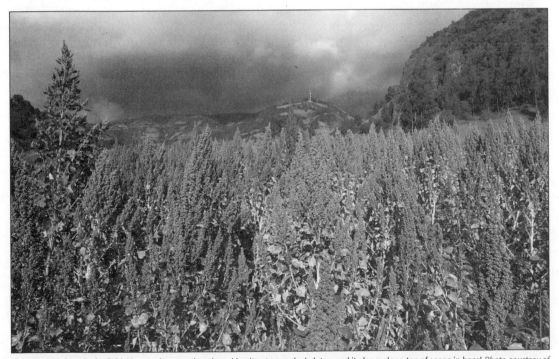

Figure 2.8. Quinoa in the field. More and more quinoa is making it onto peoples' plates, and it also makes a ton of sense in beer! *Photo courtesy of Luis Miguel Obando Tobón.*

in particular β-glucan. I still see this grain as analogous to a character malt because of the unique flavor it elicits. It is also one of the more expensive items you can add to a gluten-free grain bill, so you tend to find it relegated to a supporting role in commercial gluten-free beers.

Buckwheat. Buckwheat is now easy to source raw as groats or roasted as "kasha," as well as in malted form, with pale malts and some caramel/crystal and roasted malts available. Buckwheat found at the grocery store is typically dehusked and light in color. Although malted buckwheat appears black, you will not extract color from the husk of this grain (as is also true for sunflower seeds).

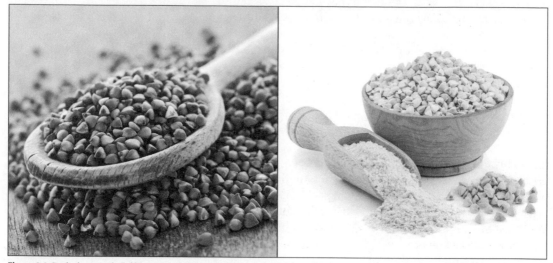

Figure 2.9. Buckwheat seeds (left) have a dark hull. Buckwheat groats (right) are light in color once the hull has been removed.
© Getty/Elenathewise (seeds); AndreyGorulko (groats)

Freshly ground buckwheat often lends a noticeable nutty aroma and taste, and when malted and featured in a beer seems to lend a spicy and oftentimes peppery flavor—I describe its flavor as a cross between black pepper and clove, but it can be slightly earthy or vegetal at times. Buckwheat roast malts can provide great astringency and richness, and some of the crystal or caramel versions of this malt can often bring flavors of chocolate, toasted biscuit, and toffee.

Buckwheat is most prized for its ability to increase head retention, body, and lacing; the malted form yields 28 PPG (234 °l/kg). It can also aid greatly in mouthfeel even with low finishing gravities, something many other gluten-free grains struggle to do. Recent research suggests that buckwheat has β-amylase (although α-amylase is almost non-existent), making it a great pairing with a grain like millet, which possesses complimentary α-amylase (Ledley et al. 2021, 13).

Amaranth. Amaranth can be found malted, but is more commonly available raw. I do not have much experience with this grain living in North America, but most sources focus on its nutty taste. It is quite small in size (even more so than millet or sorghum, which are small themselves), so there are false bottom considerations when lautering, as well as milling considerations—assuming you can get your gap settings tight enough, the friability is there but make sure you crush up enough endosperm for starch conversion.

ADDITIONAL ADJUNCTS
Hey, since we're already in the deep end, let's get whacky! While all gluten-free fermentables are, by a barley brewer's definition, considered "adjuncts," the ingredients that follow are a bit farther afield even for brewers of gluten-free beer.

Chestnuts. Chestnuts can be found both dried and roasted. Breweries like Ground Breaker have found that chesnuts can help add maltiness to the finished product and they can be roasted in-house to various levels in order to produce great dark beers. In fact, Ground Breaker's Dark Ale is one of the most decorated dark gluten-free beers. Chestnuts also have a long history in Italian beers, including a style called *birra alle castagne* (literally "chestnut beer"). Unlike many other tree nuts, chestnuts are low in fat, but they are also high in carbohydrates, which is good for making beer as they will not disrupt head retention like many other tree nuts do.

Given that many people who need a gluten-free diet also have tree nut allergies, please use these (and all tree nuts) with caution.

Tapioca. I have personally only found tapioca in extract form (powdered maltodextrin and syrup). By all accounts, it does not really offer much flavor contribution at all. Tapioca extract could be ideal when trying to dry a beer out or increase the gravity. In its maltodextrin form, tapioca can lend unfermentable material to add body to the mouthfeel of a finished beer.

Sunflower seeds. Commonly available raw, sunflower seeds are also available malted; however, these "malts" come from facilities that also malt and process barley and wheat products, so use with extreme caution. The malted seeds have a noteworthy nutty taste, and I would recommend using them in smaller quantities, depending on the style.

Lentils. I have noticed a slight vegetal taste from lentils, if any taste. The main use for lentils is to provide body and head retention due to their massive quantity of protein by weight. A quarter pound of lentils in a five-gallon batch (just 6 g per liter) can go a long way. Lentils can also be roasted, which not only adds color but also exposes more carbohydrate material in the lentils so some fermentable sugars are extracted in the mash as well, although nowhere near that of other grains and extracts.

Sweet potatoes. While sweet potatoes contain their own enzymes (both α- and β-amylases) this tuber only provides about 8 PPG (67 l°/kg), so you will need to use a lot. Most all-sweet potato recipes say to use more than 15 lb. for five gallons (360 g/L) if you want to get above 2.5% ABV. Additionally—and this is the case when brewing with any root vegetable—it is highly recommended to grate sweet potatoes or find a way to make the starches as aqueous as possible (such as boiling them and mashing them or even roasting them on high in the oven), as they do not have

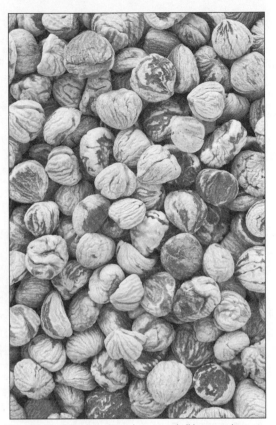

Figure 2.10. Dried chestnuts. Not just a tasty holiday treat, chestnuts are a great addition to any beer recipe. © *Getty/FotografiaBasica*

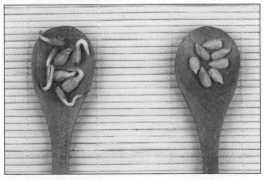

Figure 2.11. Sprouting sunflower seed. © *Getty/ogichobanov*

the same friability as a grain or pseudocereal. The skins appear to contain the highest levels of enzymes so be sure to keep them when using fresh sweet potatoes. Sweet potato flakes allow the brewer to avoid a lot of this work and are an excellent addition to your arsenal of ingredients (if you can find them easily), specifically because they are pre-gelatinized.

Given their relatively high enzyme levels, sweet potatoes can be used in conjunction with grain or other fermentables to aid in the breakdown of all starches in the mash to fermentable sugars, though you may still need to incorporate something extra for body. Another reason to use these in conjunction with grains is that sweet potatoes do not provide much in terms of head retention. In fact, sweet potatoes and other tubers and sugar products really don't have enough inherent protein to contribute to head retention.

White potato. I most commonly see white potatoes used to make vodka, but potatoes have their uses in certain beer styles. They can help to dry out a beer and they have a pretty high carbohydrate content, with flaked white potato yielding 30 PPG (250 l°/kg) on the low end and 42 PPG (350 l°/kg) on the high end. I recommend using flaked potato, as the starch will be more readily available and the mash will require much less work. As with sweet potatoes, fresh is still an option, you will just have to use a lot more since the extract yield is only 8 PPG (67 l°/kg). I advise against a 100% white potato beer as this vegetable does not really contribute any flavor or other beer-like elements, but it can help boost the starting OG. It performs best as a base ingredient or paired with other ingredients that lend more character.

Cassava. Cassava is another low-flavor option more commonly used in the production of spirits, but these tubers only yield about 11.5 PPG (96 l°/kg) when used whole. I recommend the syrup extract over whole cassava for that reason.

Belgian candi syrup/sugar. Belgian candi syrups/sugars are made from sugars refined from beets. Whole beets themselves have a low carbohydrate content by weight and yield just ~2 PPG (~17 l°/kg). The candi syrups, however, can contribute about 32 PPG (267 l°/kg) and can help boost your starting gravity. Candi syrups and sugars range in taste from neutral (clear/light) to dark caramel (dark/amber). They are used to provide clean fermentables that dry out the beer, possibly providing some color. They can contribute a pretty prominent flavor depending on your grain bill, especially the darker versions. Some darker versions also contain date sugar.

Molasses. Not commonly seen in beers nowadays, this is still a lovely ingredient in certain styles. Molasses was a feature of some old homebrew recipes, and has even found its way into some recent commercial beers, like Freedom Reserve Red Lager that Anheuser-Busch released in 2018. It can be featured up to about 10% of a recipe, but higher quantities might contribute an off-putting metallic flavor in the finished beer. Interestingly enough, dry yeast producers commonly use molasses in their propagating media, so in essence any beer made with these yeasts technically contains molasses.

UNEXPECTED TREASURE TROVES

I understand that many people who are reading this may not possess the budget to have gluten-free malts shipped to them wherever they are in the world. However, there are so many places that sell gluten-free grains and other fermentables, you just have to have your radar tuned in.

Health food stores have a vast variety! Bulk bins have some incredible finds: from lentils to chestnuts, from quinoa to millet, and from dried mushrooms to herbs. You can create some truly amazing beers with ingredients found just down the street. Imagine styles and tastes that are only slightly outside of the box.

So what if the grains are not malted? Partial mash anyone? Maybe you cannot get sorghum, but you probably could get agave, corn syrup, honey, rice syrup, or cane sugar; and do not forget maple syrup. You can toast unmalted grains to your liking for character and color. You can even caramelize those extracts and syrups even further in darker styles to bring out deeper and richer flavors.

This is where having a fundamentally curious spirit helps, but your preferences will determine your go-to base recipe. Some prejudice has developed against the metallic/green apple flavor note that sorghum elicits, and while its historic use among gluten-free brewers has contributed to the preconception of a "gluten-free flavor," that does not mean you should treat sorghum as an inferior ingredient. Just make sure you add enough nutrients for the fermentation, and most yeasts will make you wonderful tasting beers. Sorghum can be found in African and American grocery stores alike and is a great base malt. Making a drink like umqombothi—a traditional African beer, made with sorghum, and oftentimes corn as well, consumed locally and in traditional ceremonies across Africa—is a lot easier to consider now.

SEED COMPANIES AND FARM SUPPLY

Seed companies and farm suppliers will definitely have what you want if you are looking for whole grain sorghum, millet, quinoa, buckwheat, lentils, etc. But your minimum buy may be slightly higher, so I recommend this source mostly to people who have ample storage space and the wherewithal to malt and/or roast these grains for beer making. Since you are buying direct and with minimal process, the price per pound is cheaper, which is still a worthy consideration.

MAKING YOUR OWN MALT

Malting is a process by which a maltster begins the germination process with the seed, essentially telling it to "grow a plant," and then ending that process a few days later through drying and roasting. The main reason to malt is to generate enzymatic activity within the grain kernel that will then be used to degrade starches in the mash process to create wort. These enzymes would otherwise be used by the seed to convert the internal starches to food that is used to grow into a plant, but by prematurely stopping the germination process the maltster saves this resource for the brewer.

There are some specific steps that need to be taken by the would-be maltster to create clean and safe malts to brew with. If you are looking to malt at home, Gluten Free Home Brewing (https://www.glutenfreehomebrewing.com) has several tutorials in its resources section aimed at the beginner and more advanced levels. In addition, useful information about malting procedures can be gleaned from peer-reviewed papers relating to brewing research; for example, the methods section of Ledley et al. (2021, sec. 2.2). I cannot claim any expertise in the area of home-malting, as I have not yet attempted to do it, but please do not let my ignorance on the topic dissuade you from creating your own home-malting program. The resources are out there to help you achieve your goal of making world-class gluten-free beer. The best advice I can offer on the topic of home-malting is to control elements like black mold as these will render your end product non-viable in the brewhouse.

A PREFACE ON RECIPE FORMULATION

ENTERING COMPETITIONS

There are always reasons to get an expert's opinion on your creations, if your ego can take it. When it comes to many judges, while their palates are understandably not attuned to these gluten-free grains, they know which flavors mean what, especially when it comes to infections. Special consideration of grains/fermentables is necessary if you are trying to produce beers that meet the definitions of traditional barley-based beer styles. For example, a 100% sorghum beer will typically have a noticeable flavor, while a similar recipe with millet would "pass" more easily in such a style.

Judges have fantastic, discerning palates, and many judges seem to be able to pick out ingredients like sorghum nowadays. However, if you nail your beer category with the correct flavors, aromas, and overall quality, you have a shot at the podium, even in barley-based categories. Dedicated gluten-free Holidaily Brewing Company has had success competing against barley-based beers and it's especially noteworthy that gluten-free brewers have done well with lagers, which can be some of the most unforgiving categories. I have entered into barley-dominated categories to see how close I can come to the style: at the 2017 Los Angeles County Fair I placed third in the IPA category with a gluten-free beer.

> Sometimes judges will give you a knee-slapper. For example, I have used millet in a recipe in the Alternative Grain category and still had judges unsure of why I would use that grain . . . they literally asked, "Why millet?" in the notes. It gets even funnier: at least a couple of commercial gluten-free brewers have been marked down when their beer "didn't taste gluten-free."

Right off the bat, the gluten-free category is one of the hardest to judge and be judged in. It is up there with the experimental beer categories or other similar categories where drastically different base beer styles compete against each other.

If a beer displays a noticeable flaw, or there is something that draws it out of the base style indicated by the competitor, there is little chance at earning a medal in competition. In fact, there have been years where only two medals have been awarded in the gluten-free category at the GABF, even with over 45 entries. That means every single one of the other entries had some clear flaw that kept them from the podium. Many gluten-free grains just cannot be considered when trying to make a "true-to-style" product. For example, oats are extremely unlikely to produce a true-to-style Vienna lager, for example, but oats do make sense in a stout or hazy IPA. This is where going the extra mile and spending that extra buck for the malts and ingredients that make a better representation of a style make a massive difference.

There seem to be certain flavors (spice, specifically) that may throw some barley-beer drinkers off. You may run into difficulties when using any grains that produce spicy flavors. Buckwheat is a good example: you will likely need to incorporate buckwheat in some capacity if you wish to make something reminiscent of a style known for its head retention, specifically lagers, which are known for lacing the whole way down the glass. When I create a recipe, I would not necessarily say that I have one grain in my kit that can do everything. In fact, I would recommend blending various malts in any true-to-style clone you are attempting.

GLUTEN-FREE BEER CAN BE ITS OWN THING

Long-standing conventions in beer naming have made the conversation of brewing clones with gluten-free grains an interesting one. Consider a style like Pilsner for example. Not using a Pilsner malt, a key ingredient for a style like this, makes recreating a gluten-free "Pilsner" seem almost a non-starter, but this has spawned some fun takes: Divine Science trademarked the name "Millsner" (millet Pilsner) for this very reason. In theory, you could make a "Silsner" (sorghum) or "Rilsner" (rice), and I know many a beer philosopher would agree that those names are more fitting than trying to use "Pilsner" purely out of historical respect for the naming conventions that exist for barley-based beer.

The future for gluten-free beer is getting brighter and brighter. There is now an annual BJCP-sanctioned competition in Golden, CO hosted by Holidaily Brewing Company, and also competitions hosted by some members of the Zero Tolerance Gluten Free Homebrewing Club.

On a larger scale, the inclusion of gluten-free brewing in the barley and wheat-dominated world of beer production will allow for the expansion of many beer drinkers' palates, not to mention encourage more focus on locality, purpose, and sustainability. Which brings me to my next thought: since it is not the same, why be the same? Nothing trumps locality, especially when it comes to ingredients native to a specific climate. For some, rice is much easier to find than millet; in some countries, amaranth and teff are much easier to source than buckwheat or sorghum. No matter where you are, there are beers to be made! If this sense of place is manifested in a beer produced from local ingredients, I see no reason why it always has to include barley or even taste like a beer made from barley.

GENERAL CONSIDERATIONS FOR BREWING GLUTEN FREE

When thinking about beer, there are some highly important elements that people expect. Here are some general points to keep in mind when setting out to make a world-class gluten-free beer. Use the following as a way to imagine yourself inside the mind of a beer judge:

- **Taste:** Are all the right grain and adjunct flavors present for the given style referenced? Additionally, are all the right style-specific hop and yeast derived flavors present on the palate?
- **Mouthfeel:** Is the thickness or thinness on the palate appropriate given the name or style being referenced in your gluten-free beer? Does the given style call for a higher residual sugar content or does it call for a drier experience?
- **Aroma:** Does your beer put off the correct beer aromas for the style referenced? Does the given style call for hop- or yeast-derived aromas, or does it require grain-forward smells?
- **Finish:** Do the appropriate aromas, mouthfeel, and flavors dissipate, or linger into a memorable and world-class experience for the drinker?

Our focus will be all these aspects when designing recipes as we progress through the coming chapters. These will affect our grain and adjunct selection, as well as the enzymes we choose—recent research has shown that various enzymes and mash regimes can potentially yield very different beers, even when the same grain bill is used. There are certain brewing outcomes that others have experienced that I cannot recreate myself, and more research is needed to truly unpack all the truths about these gluten-free grains and adjuncts and their use in the brewhouse. For example, Ledley et al. (2021, 16) shows how a modified mash with malted teff produces highly fermentable wort comparable to that from a barley-based infusion mash. From the experiences that have been shared with me by other gluten-free brewers, most actually recommend staying away from teff specifically due to its incredibly small grain size, which leads to difficulties with false bottoms and lautering, with most brewers experiencing stuck mashes. Thus, there seems to be a gap at the academic level from what is happening in the actual brewhouse, which poses some interesting questions.

I am sure there are many studies like the one by Ledley et al. waiting to be done at the academic research level that will demonstrate the viability of these grains. Further investment in research is needed if we are to map the true beer-making potential of all the grains mentioned in this chapter and beyond. For now, however, there are some incredible flavors available to explore further in chapter 3.

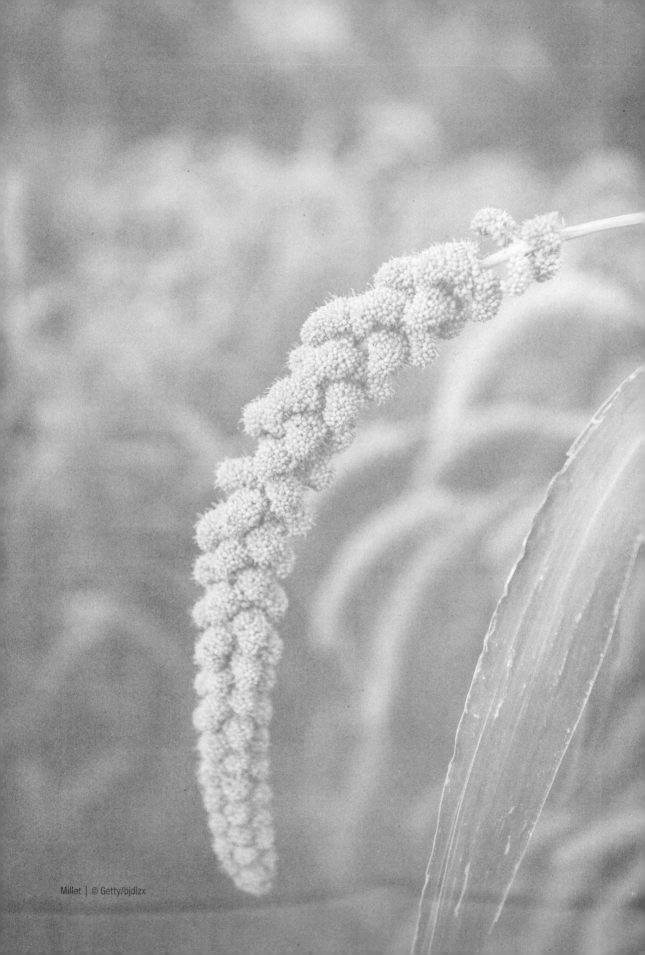

3

Base and Character Malts and Adjuncts

e took a high-level look at the kinds of malt and other fermentables available to gluten-free brewers in the previous chapter, but that's just establishing a baseline. At this point we are almost ready to start creating recipes, so it's important to know what is really available out there. I am most familiar with US-based maltsters that specialize in gluten-free products, and I will dig into those at length here. Many of the grains and adjuncts mentioned here are available all over the world; while there may be variances due to local growing conditions or practices, these grains and adjuncts have general properties that remain fairly consistent. However, I cannot guarantee whether they are available in other parts of the world in all the forms discussed here (malts, roasts, extracts, etc.). When creating a grain bill, it is important to note the specific varietal (e.g., proso millet versus German millet) as this can have a substantial impact on the brewing properties of the grain or adjunct.

Certain gluten-free pale malts, crystal malts, and roast malts have different starch and sugar contents when matched up against their barley-based counterparts. Another important difference is the need to use additional (exogenous) enzymes when mashing with many gluten-free grains and adjuncts. The combination of these has led to the common thinking that gluten-free grains produce drier beers than those made with conventional grains. The starch content of certain grains like glutinous rice and waxy maize is almost 100% amylopectin. The corn from Grouse Malting is dent corn, which typically contains up to 30% amylose by weight but still contains a high level of amylopectin. Both rice and corn (maize) contain starches that are great precursors for sugar, but these cereals contain almost no amylase enzymes. In other words, rice and corn have low to zero diastatic power, so they are great for sugar extraction and fermentation when used with exogenous enzymes. However, even with added enzymes, if these fermentables are used exclusively in this type of mash regimen, or with the wrong type of enzymes (specifically glucoamylases and glucosidases), the resulting high-glucose wort that can be created from a starch like amylopectin results in a beer that is overattenuated, having a thin cider-like body. With a low finishing gravity and lower protein content, there could also be less beer foam stability on top of that. Of course, if you do not use any exogenous enzymes with grains such as rice and corn, your wort will not be fermentable at all! The techniques that we will explore in chapter 5 will show how these gluten-free grains can be used and keep the resulting product completely within style boundaries.

Some of the following flavors and roasts of malts are still proprietary to dedicated gluten-free malthouses like Grouse Malt House and Eckert Malting and Brewing Co., but there are several that I have seen available from multiple suppliers. Traditional barley malthouses such as Skagit Valley Malting, Colorado Malting Company, and various others have started to add gluten-free base and character malts like millet, buckwheat, and sorghum. Many of these traditional malthouses use shared equipment, though some have dedicated equipment for gluten-free grains. I always recommend calling ahead to these businesses, as some share the same mills between glutenous and gluten-free grains, but now have dedicated malt beds and kilns. However, cross contamination is always a concern so it is worth being cautious. Many of the non-dedicated facilities do not currently qualify for a "gluten-free" label due to these concerns, and many commercial brewers do not use them to ensure consumer safety (this is at time of publishing). It should also be noted that some maltsters, like Eckert, have chosen to not renew their gluten-free certifications because their standards already exceed the requirements listed by certifying bodies, being that they are dedicated facilities that buy from producers whose products never interact with ingredients that contain gluten.

HOT STEEP EVALUATION

If you would like to follow along at home as we review fermentables and their tastes, you can use the American Society of Brewing Chemists (ASBC) Hot Steep Malt Evaluation Method to evaluate them.* To begin, procure your desired malt or adjunct, crush the grains to a flour-like consistency, and then allow the grist to steep in hot water for around 10–15 minutes; after steeping, separate the grains from the water using a funnel and filter. Once the resulting solution is at a drinkable temperature, you can note the flavor contributions of the grains.

* ASBC Methods of Analysis (online), "Sensory Analysis 14. Hot Steep Malt Sensory Evaluation Method," approved 2017 (St. Paul, MN: American Society of Brewing Chemists), doi: 10.1094/ASBCMOA-Sensory Analysis-14 (subscription required); Cassie Poirier, "The Hot Steep Method: Step-by-Step Instructions," Briess Malt & Ingredients Co., March 26, 2019, https://www.brewingwithbriess.com/blog/the-hot-steep-method-step-by-step-instructions/.

COLOR RATINGS

Where appropriate, the color of malts and adjuncts is given in degrees Lovibond (°L) as this is still the unit most prevalent in the US malting industry. For the most part, degrees Lovibond are equivalent to Standard Reference Method (SRM) points used to denote the color of beer. For European Brewery Convention (EBC) units of color measurement, the conversion is EBC = SRM × 1.97, or one EBC unit is approximately twice the degrees Lovibond or SRM reading.

SORGHUM

Whether you are using malted grain or unmalted extract, sorghum (1–9°L) seems to create beers that are more cider-like than people typically expect. Most commonly, BriesSweet™ White Sorghum Extract has historically dominated taste expectations for would-be tasters and brewers of gluten-free beer, though with the rise of new malts and adjuncts this perception is rapidly changing. There are some *malted* red sorghum liquid extracts (i.e., sorghum LME) that have recently become available that lend what the average brewer would call a "cleaner" taste; however, they are not as easy to find (I have only ever seen red sorghum LME on Gluten Free Brew Supply's website).

The widespread appeal of the BriesSweet™ extract product has resulted in an interesting paradigm for brewers of gluten-free beer, at least in the US. This sorghum extract is highly accessible domestically at fairly reasonable prices, and it has great extract potential; but it can lend some questionable characteristics when used as a base fermentable, a sorghum extract "twang" that is described as a metallic and bitter malt character. This problem can be mitigated with the use of ample yeast nutrient: the secret being the use of high-FAN yeast nutrient as opposed to B vitamin–heavy nutrients. When using any extract as the base fermentable, there tends to be a lack of fullness and malt character in the final beer—extract beers are often considered "lacking" in some of these essential qualities when compared to all-grain brews, regardless of whether it is a gluten-free brew or not.

Additionally, many all-malt sorghum beers finish quite dry, suggesting that mashing sorghum malts produces a wort high in glucose and maltose. I have regularly seen sorghum malt-based beers with a final gravity (FG) between 1.001 and 1.005 (0.3–1.3°P).

FREE AMINO NITROGEN

Free amino nitrogen (FAN) is defined as the sum of the individual amino acids, ammonium ions, and small peptides (di- and tripeptides) in wort, which constitute the sources of nitrogen that yeast can assimilate during fermentation. Some brewing scientists regard FAN as a better predictor than wort sugars of healthy yeast growth, viability, vitality, fermentation efficiency, and hence beer quality and stability.[*] Even if attenuation of wort sugars proceeds normally, production of the same quality of beer is not always guaranteed if FAN levels are too low or too high, suggesting that attenuation alone is not a good indicator of yeast performance.

[*] Graham G. Stewart, "free amino nitrogen (FAN)," The Oxford Companion to Beer definition, Craft Beer & Brewing, Accessed May 2, 2022, https://beerandbrewing.com/dictionary/o1j9KOtQ4v/ .

Using extra yeast food with sorghum malt or syrup is best practice but you can run the risk of drying out your beer. I recommend the right kind of mash regime and enzyme dosage to finish with the right beer-like qualities in all-malt sorghum beers (see chapter 5), and adding some sort of dextrin ingredient (like maltodextrin) in the boil to make sure you have the right finishing gravity no matter what yeast you choose.

Co-allergen alert!
Please note that some yeast nutrient preparations possess ingredients like dairy and soy. These are potential allergens, and many people who have a gluten allergy are also allergic to dairy and soy.

Sorghum can provide different flavors and characters to those found in barley-based beers, typically tart green apple or slight citrus notes, and possibly a malty bitterness or astringency. While these are considered off-flavors for barley, they are part of the character of sorghum and can be embraced as a way of providing new dimensionality to your brews. Given the citrusy-apple notes, sorghum can lend cider or wine-like (think sauvignon blanc) flavors that do well in blonde ales, American lagers, fruited beers, IPAs, farmhouse ales, and saisons. This flavor profile combined with the dryness from sorghum beer's typical low finishing gravity makes this grain well-suited to producing drinkable and quenching beers that seem light, even when above 7% ABV.

Brewers have claimed to be able to get north of 33 PPG (275 l°/kg) from sorghum, which is certainly possible with malted sorghum when using exogenous enzymes. Without added enzymes, expect around 27–29 PPG (225–242 l°/kg) reliably (using the method discussed in chapter 5). Red or white sorghum extract will typically lend about 35 PPG (292 l°/kg), whether from malted or unmalted sources. Like millet (discussed below), the magic temperature for all-grain mashing with sorghum malt seems to be above the denaturing temperature of endogenous α-amylase, at around 175°F (around 79°C) where the starches fully gelatinize.

I have not been able to find sorghum (unmalted or malted) in any other varieties besides white and red. Red sorghum makes a deeper colored mash that turns golden to yellow in the boil; so, either way, you will come out with a fizzy yellow beverage whichever you choose. When you want to add character, I suggest one or more of the grains that are described in this chapter. That being said, you can roast sorghum grain yourself, and you can still make many styles using sorghum extract or malted sorghum as your primary fermentable.

RICE

I recommend using syrups when starting out with rice as well, which is why rice follows sorghum in this discussion; for example, the best pairing for a beginner is to use roughly 50:50 sorghum syrup and brown rice syrup. You can expect good extract potential from rice extracts and syrups, around 37 PPG (309 l°/kg), as well as additional amino acids that contribute to FAN. But the true beauty of rice comes in using whole grains, and not just for drainage. As you progress with gluten-free brewing, rice syrup solids should really be looked at as more of an adjunct (unless you are making a hopped seltzer, I guess). There is such a wonderfully diverse set of flavors that rice and rice malts can contribute to beer and they can be featured in any recipe you choose to make.

Calrose rice, unmalted (0°L). A medium-grain white rice most commonly seen in sushi and other Japanese dishes, Calrose rice forms the bulk of the California rice crop. Despite its easy availability, I would wait to tackle Calrose rice until you have some gluten-free brews under your belt. In particular, you should nail down how to use exogenous enzymes and learn how well your mash equipment drains gluten-free grains, otherwise you could unwittingly create more problems for yourself than is really needed as you are just getting into it. Hey, at least you might end up with a bowl of rice.

Once you have a couple of brews under your belt and you are looking for a cheeky way to spend less money, Calrose rice is a great grain to have in your arsenal. Medium-grain white rice typically does not need proteases or rice hulls (although they can help), and the flavor is rich and crisp all at the same time. Maybe you've had a Japanese rice lager before, so you're likely no stranger to that wonderful taste that helps lighten a beer without compromising flavor.

Basmati rice (0°L). A great brewing grain, specifically because basmati rice's starch reserves are more readily accessible than Calrose. Using only α-amylase will likely do the trick with this grain. When you inspect basmati rice under a microscope, you see that it has many small starch granules that expand with heat and burst to leave soluble starch chains that can be cleaved into sugars easily by the added enzymes.

Instant rice (0°L). Instant rice is likely one of the superior store-bought rice varieties you can buy for brewing, specifically because it is precooked and, thus, pregelatinized. Being pregelatinized means instant rice will be even more effective than basmati, as the starch grains are readily available for an exogenous α-amylase.

Black rice, a.k.a. "Forbidden Rice" (2.5°L). Although the smell is akin to that of Calrose or basmati rice, black rice types are different cultivars and can appear coal black. Black rice turns the mash purple, though a drop in acidity from boiling, hop additions, or yeast activity will rapidly shift this to a nice yellow. In all honesty, when black rice is used in a beer it is likely for marketing effect, as I have not noticed much difference from other rice varieties, only the higher price in the grocery aisle. If you are using high quantities of other rices like Calrose, basmati, or instant rice, then black rice could technically help lend some color, but my suggestion for that is to use at least one of the forms of malted rice discussed in the next section.

MALTED RICE

Rice malts are necessary to get all the flavors and textures you are looking for in a beer, and they are worth the money spent. Rice is one of the most affordable malted grains you can buy for gluten-free brewing at this time. However, typical rice malts may not supply all you need, specifically enough protein content to create good foam, although many newly available enzymes seem to help with head and lacing in rice beers. I would use at least 40% rice malt when making rice beers to help with reliability and consistency in your brews (typically, millet would make up the rest of the grain bill, although you could use 30% buckwheat or quinoa). Additionally, rice malts can provide flavors that better reflect barley-based beer than unmalted rice, and they are less likely to have issues with starches making their way into the boil and subsequently into the beer. Along with previously noted issues with low FAN and yeast nutrients in rice, this is potentially another reason for the off-flavors like celery and wintergreen that have been noted with beers made with rice. Additional yeast nutrient is still needed to prevent such flavors, but unmalted rice is more likely to develop these specific off-flavors due to the increased starches in boil.

At time of publication, there was only one rice maltster and roaster in the world producing at the commercial level, Eckert Malting and Brewing, in Chico, CA. The following is a discussion of their current products.

Pale rice malt (3°L). The pale rice malt is a great base malt with a neutral taste and can be featured in any recipe. Brewers often use this grain as the main fermentable because of its extract potential (31 PPG, or 259 l°/kg) and it provides great drainage in the mash. It lends a slight straw and biscuit aroma and a crisp tingle on the palate. Since rice is similar to sorghum in that it needs a good clean fermentation to taste its best, pale rice malt (and rice malt in general) can give a noticeable phenolic spice or wintergreen flavor, which can be mitigated by maintaining proper yeast health.

De-hulled pale rice malt (1°L). I like to call de-hulled pale rice malt my "brewhouse beast." Since rice is so much hull by weight and surface area, the de-hulled rice malt has the same flavor as pale rice malt with almost 30% more extract potential, bringing de-hulled pale rice malt's extract potential up to 40 PPG (334 l°/kg). At time of writing, this product is readily available for commercial brewers but not typically for homebrewers (although Eckert's "Gas Hog" is, which is a de-hulled, roasted rice malt, discussed below). If your recipe already features rice with hulls, then de-hulled pale rice malt is a great way to increase the gravity of your wort. You will likely get a bit less color than from pale rice malt with hulls, but color nonetheless.

Biscuit rice malt (5°L). The 5°L biscuit rice malt is a great addition to any recipe, with a biscuity-malt taste that is true to its name. When used in the right quantity, this malt has gotten me quite close to a "barley" flavor.

Biscuit rice malt (15°L). The 15°L biscuit rice malt has much more of a bread crust or toast flavor and aroma, with a slight color addition; great for pale, blonde, and even amber ales, as well as all sorts of lager styles. It does have a bit less residual sweetness than some of the other biscuit rice malts, making it ideal for adding complexity without additional sugars.

Biscuit rice malt (18°L). The 18°L biscuit rice malt gives off a dark bread or pumpernickel aroma and taste. The flavor is much more potent than the color in this grain suggests and can provide complexity to a lot of styles.

Dark biscuit rice malt (28°L). The dark biscuit rice malt can provide a slight umami flavor (similar notes to brown rice-green tea, or *genmaicha*). Although umami might sound a little unusual when describing a malt, it can be desirable in many beer styles. The *sencha*-esque, or green-tea, character from the astringency of the roast essentially delivers that characteristic umami, and the *genmai* note is the toasty, warm nuttiness that comes typically from the popped rice used to make the tea, but this flavor in dark biscuit rice malt it is due to the roasting technique used by Eckert. A truly complex experience, this flavor profile lends itself to a smoked IPA, stout, porter, rauchbier, schwarzbier, or Belgian dubbel and easily so many more.

> *Something to note when doing pre-mash flavor tests: no matter how hot you steep rice malt, you likely will not get much sugar when you make your grain tea (due to the lack of enzymatic activity), though you will get a feel for the aroma and color of the malt.*

Amber rice malt (15°L). Visually, amber rice malt does not appear to be much different than the 15°L version of biscuit rice malt, but this amber malt can add great color and a toasted, sweet bread note to all sorts of styles, even when used in small quantities, and especially in lagers. I have used amber rice malt for up to 50% of the grain bill and have gotten great results without having the beer be overly sweet, but I have even seen some anecdotes that suggest it can be used at 80% or more of the grain bill. It is available de-hulled as well.

Crystal rice malt (16°L). Crystal rice malt has a rich sweetness with a slight caramel/honey note. This malt is my go-to grain for West Coast IPAs, pale ales, and any other style you want to give a slight ruddy tint to. This is another malt that you can use for up to 50% of the grain bill without it dominating the flavor too much. Crystal rice malt also comes in de-hulled form.

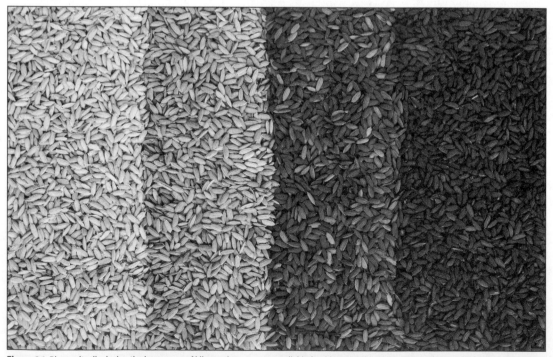

Figure 3.1. Rice malts displaying the large array of kilns and roasts now available for this grain. This variety means you could theoretically make most beer styles with just rice if you so choose, assuming you use an appropriate mash regimen (see chap. 5).

James' Brown Rice malt (22°L). The James' Brown Rice malt from Eckert contributes notes of spicy chocolate and caramel. It lends itself to British-style ales, dark lagers, and Belgian-style ales with its unique character and flavor contributions. This malt is especially well-suited for gluten-free brown ales. James' Brown Rice also comes in de-hulled form.

Dark rice malt (150°L). Another great go-to for darker styles, dark rice malt provides lovely notes of coffee, chocolate, and burnt or over-roasted genmai. You might need to use more than 10% dark rice malt in the grain bill to get appreciable color from it. I have had stout recipes turn out more like an amber or red ale because I overestimated the color contribution dark rice malt would provide.

"Gas Hog" rice malt (350-400°L). Eckert's "Gas Hog" rice malt is aptly named, as it is left in the roaster long enough to develop a very dark color. In fact, some of the first batches that Eckert produced would ignite upon exiting the kiln. Gas Hog is definitely a character malt that belongs in stouts and porters, providing some color to the foam along with rich cacao and coffee notes. However, be careful with your mash pH as this malt can add a fair amount of acidity—your target mash pH should be between 4.9 and 5.9 depending on the enzymes you are using. On top of that, be conscious of your fermentability, as you may lose much of the richness if your resulting beer dries out too far. You will be left with a product that can be overly bitter or astringent to the point of unpleasant . . . I have picked up ash notes or "soggy campfire" before. This very dark malt needs to be balanced with unmalted grains and crystal malts to help with residual sweetness. Gas Hog is one of the best grains to purchase in its de-hulled form: the best strategy is to use 50:50 with-hulls and de-hulled forms to get its full flavor potential. Usually, you will not be using enough of this grain to care about sugar extract from it, so you may choose to add this malt after a higher temperature gelatinization step has already occurred if you are worried about pulling too many husk tannins.

> *Rice is not the only grain that can technically ignite after it exits the kiln, but there are some factors that mean rice is prone to doing so. The fat content of the grain can be close to scorching or flash temperatures in the roaster, which is a closed atmosphere devoid of oxygen. As it exits the roaster, exposure to an oxygen-rich environment and a high enough temperature combines with friction between grain fibers to cause combustion. Something to consider for any would-be rice maltster.*

Pitch Black rice malt (400+°L). Introduced by Eckert in 2020, Pitch Black rice malt is roasted to provide dark, robust coffee and raw cacao chocolate notes. Even at 0.2%–0.5% of the grain bill, this malt will almost guarantee a darker beer; in such small quantities people can still pick up some maple and fudge notes. Pitch Black is what some might call gluten-free's answer to black patent malt. It has truly changed the game for brewing with rice—it was assumed rice could not achieve this deep of a color. But now the future is dark, baby, real dark.

MILLET

Millet is now available in malted and raw versions, with various crystals and roasted malts all the way up to 260°L. This is a grain that some call "Old Faithful" for a reason—a diverse flavor profile and extraction rates that you can rely on when using a multitude of different enzymes. As I alluded to in chapter 2, you don't technically *need* exogenous enzymes when using millet, but they do help a great deal when striving to make world-class beer, as well as with getting your money's worth. Proso millet specifically has been researched as a commercially viable substitute for barley (Zarnkow et al. 2010; Ledley et al. 2021).

For brewers in the US, the most commonly available millet varieties are white proso and red proso, with white proso being the most common of the two. Due to the higher friability of these

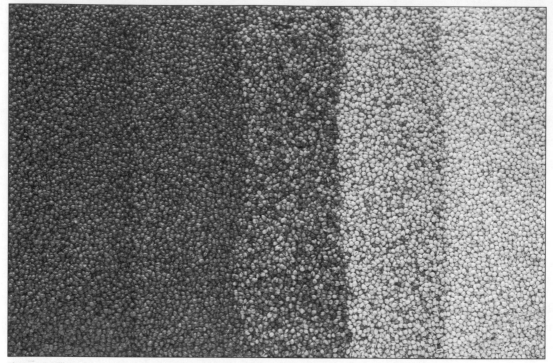

Figure 3.2. Millet malts now come in an impressive range of colors and flavors. The number of specialty millet malts is increasing all the time—between writing this book to its final edit, Grouse Malt House enlarged its range of millet malts by about 30%.

grains compared to other species of millet (Japanese millet and foxtail, or German, millet), proso millet can, in my opinion, be used exclusively to make just about any beer.

At time of writing, Grouse Malt House in Wellington, CO is the main dedicated gluten-free producer of millet malts in the US. Therefore, the ensuing descriptions of millet malts will focus on those types produced by Grouse.

Raw, conventional, millet seed, or unmalted millet (1°L). Unmalted millet is one of the undiscovered gems in the gluten-free brewing world. Although it does not pack as much of a flavor punch as its malted counterpart, unmalted millet can be used for up to 40% of the grain bill, reliably yielding 25 PPG (209 l°/kg). It lends itself well to continental European styles because of the dextrins it leaves behind and the rocky foam it creates, akin to buckwheat. The dextrin and protein content also make it incredibly well-suited to certain styles like wheat beer and saison, and can bring extra body and haze stability to a hazy IPA. Think of unmalted millet as a "foam contributor" for your mash, because the protein molecules that contribute to foam stability do not get broken down as much as they do in malted forms. Due to this being an unmalted product, it will possess very little, if any, endogenous enzymes; this product requires the use of exogenous enzymes.

Pale millet malt (1.3–2.4°L). Pale millet malt is one of the most common base malts used in gluten-free homebrewing and is typically handled like Pilsner malt. Straightforward and to the point, with a sweet, neutral taste and straw color, it belongs in any style. After sorghum syrup extract, pale millet malt is the product that you will find most consistently in use at just about any gluten-free brewery operation.

Vienna millet malt (1.7–3.9°L). Vienna millet malt packs an immensely sweet and malty taste, with a bready aroma that builds to toffee notes when used in larger quantities. It can be used as a base malt, but most brewers will typically use Vienna millet malt at a rate below 50% of the grain bill to provide depth. This malt comes in handy for any of the malt-forward styles, like many British ales, central European lagers and ales, and darker ales and lagers.

Munich millet malt (1.3–2.8°L). Munich millet malt has wonderful biscuit and light toasted notes. In the right quantity (about 20% of the grain bill), it can add a slight caramel flavor that remains even when a fermentation finishes dry. A great versatile grain that can be used as a base malt as well. In higher quantities, this malt is known to lend toffee notes as well.

Cara Millet malt (1.7–2.8°L). Cara Millet is a malt that gives sweet caramel flavors even with 100% attenuation, great when used in American IPAs to provide a sense of sweetness in an otherwise dry beer (meaning that it can stand up to hop creep), and perfect for helping balance against bitterness. Cara Millet can also be used as a base malt, but cost might be a mitigating factor. Its tendency toward sweetness means Cara Millet makes sense in cream ales and white stouts.

Caramel millet malt (3.5–5°L). Grouse Malt House's caramel millet malt is a true testament to malt innovation. Grouse devised and executed a way to promote a truer crystal through the use of exogenous enzymes, creating a gluten-free crystal malt that promotes increased residual sugars and has a rich caramel taste. This malt can be used in just about any style that needs some caramel flavor; do not be shy just because it is a crystal malt. It runs at a higher price point, so it is best suited as a character malt.

> *I once made a beer that ended up having an acetaldehyde off-flavor, but the caramel note from the millet malt made the finished product taste like a caramel apple. We drank that beer rather quickly despite the off-flavor.*

Goldfinch Millet Malt (5.7–7.2°L). Goldfinch Millet Malt from Grouse is described as having "flavors of maple and bran, as well as toasted cereal." This is great as a character malt since it can give such a non-traditional malty flavor and aroma to any style, but especially beers with low hopping. While it can stand up against certain hops, Goldfinch Millet Malt works best in malt-forward beers to show off its flavors. Quite similar in appeal and color to Golden Promise, this malt has become my de facto malt for certain styles. Similar to Red Wing Millet (below), Goldfinch Millet Malt does not have a direct analog to a barley variety, and Grouse went with a new malt name to reflect this.

Light roast millet (11.6–15.3°L). Light roast millet is a great character malt for a soft toast, slight biscuit flavor, but also a little bit of nuttiness as well, which can work great in many styles, especially British-style ales. It can also be used in small quantities in lagers to give more depth of flavor and richness, adding something akin to the kettle caramelization often found with central European styles.

Dutch Roast millet malt (15.3–22.7°L). For a malt that is not really all that dark, there is a much larger than expected coffee taste from Dutch Roast millet malt. With a slight nuttiness, and even a little bit of chocolate, the possibilities are theoretically endless with this character malt. It works great when you want to get some roasted notes and ruby color but not all the way dark; perfect when layered in stouts and porters alike, as well as amber ales. I have even used Dutch Roast to great success in darker lager styles and coffee ambers.

Grouse Malt House had been making two flavors, American Roast and French Roast, that were almost indistinguishable from each other taste- and flavor-wise. If there was any difference, the American Roast was noted by some to have a more noticeable nuttiness than French Roast. At any rate, these two flavors became Dutch Roast millet malt. I like to say, "The French and Americans couldn't agree, so they went Dutch . . ."

Roasted Cara Millet (15.3–30.1°L). Use roasted Cara Millet malt when you want to get a rich amber color with notes of fresh baked pastries or dried fruit; some users also note hints of toffee. This is a great flavor for adding color to a hoppy amber ale or red IPA, and it is great in Belgian and British styles. This is a great character malt that does not really need any other layering unless you are going darker, such as in pastry stouts.

Red Wing millet malt (22.7–30.1°L). Lending a ruby color and notes of sweet cereal and fresh baked cookies, Red Wing millet malt is incredible when used in a pastry stout, Scotch ale, or any darker style for that matter—this malt has dark and mild ale written all over it. Red Wing is another great malt to use for color without contributing much roast flavor at all, in large part due to the process of making it—the malt is dried at a high temperature but is not actually roasted. Using it in high ratios in the grain bill will ensure a red-colored beer.

Medium roast millet malt (22.7–48.6°L). Grouse's medium roast millet malt is described as having notes of "caramel, biscuit, and coffee". It is great when used to texture in flavor, especially if the exogenous enzymes you are using are drying out your beer. Use this malt to get a fuller flavor without too much roastiness. A gradient of roasts is always advisable in any darker gluten-free style, especially stouts, so consider using this medium roast millet malt in conjunction with darker roasts to balance out a darker beer. This malt is also worth including in any brown ale and higher-ABV amber beers. As with all roasted malts, there is some evidence that the melanoidins produced during kilning may help in a small way with shelf stability but they are not a panacea for factors that lead to poor shelf life.

Griffin Millet malt (59.6–67° L). No, Grouse is not running out of bird names and using those of mythical creatures instead. The Griffin Millet malt is actually the last name of Zach, the person at Grouse who developed this malt variety. This malt is kilned longer than the average malt, and lends notes of "plum, toffee, caramelized sugar, and chocolate." Due to the kilning technique, this could in theory be used for flavor and enzymatic content, as the kilning does not exceed temperatures that denature all of the endogenous enzymes.

Roasted Goldfinch Millet malt (63.3–78.1°L). Grouse's Roasted Goldfinch Millet is probably one of the most essential character malts in any gluten-free brewer's armory. This malt gives off roasted brown sugar and caramel notes and can help you create some amazing beers, especially pale ales, imperial IPAs, Belgian styles, porters and stouts, and millet wines. If you like Goldfinch, you will love Roasted Goldfinch. This is the malt that many brewers look to when making Munich dunkels and bocks, though its residual sweetness makes it better suited to the latter.

The people at Grouse have started a "high dry" program, thanks to techniques they have recently been trying out in the kiln. They have been able to produce Vienna and Munich millet malts that are darker, in the region of 20°L Vienna and 40°L Munich barley malts, as well as the new Griffin Millet malt. Malts like these contribute darker colors to the resulting beer, but, due to using a kiln, they do not come with the roasty and nutty flavors that often result from the roaster.

Chocolate roast millet malt (92–115°L). Most liken the taste of chocolate roast millet malt to 70% (or darker) dark chocolate or bitter cacao nib, depending on how far the beer has been dried out through fermentation. Highly desirable for drier porters, and almost a no-brainer in stouts and brown ales, you can use this malt in all sorts of ways and you will probably be successful. I would even recommend throwing this malt in during the sparge just to add color and maybe a little bit of flavor; but a great option no matter how you choose to use it. At high levels it can give a slight "burnt" character to a beer, so start with a smaller amount and increase as desired.

Caramel 90L millet malt (85–95°L). Flavor descriptors associated with Caramel 90L are "honey, caramel, brown sugar, and sweet bread." Caramel 90L is a great malt for providing flavor, residual sweetness, and texture from its residual dextrins.

Caramel 120L millet malt (115–125°L). Caramel 120L millet malt has lovely notes of toffee, caramel, plum, and a light touch of chocolate. A darker version of Caramel 90L, this malt naturally provides more color and darker caramel flavors, as well as more unfermentable sugars. My mouth is watering thinking of all the ways I could use this malt. Imagine, if you will, the thought of Grouse's Caramel 120L millet malt paired with Eckert Malting's James' Brown Rice malt in a Belgian dubbel; or even with a saison yeast, or maybe in a black IPA . . . the possibilities are endless.

> *Given that gluten-free brewing typically makes use of exogenous enzymes, which tend to create more fermentable worts than their barley counterparts, Grouse's caramel malts can help you approach traditional styles without the resulting beers being overly dry.*

Dark roasted millet malt (222–260°L). I use dark roasted millet malt any time I need a roasted chocolate/coffee taste. This malt also produces a deeper beige/brown foam when used in the right quantities. Before Caramel 240L (see next) was available, the dark roasted millet malt was considered absolutely necessary when making specific gluten-free stouts "to-style."

Caramel 240L millet malt (222–245°L). From the first time I used Caramel 240L, I was sold. It has such an incredible bouquet of "sweet chocolate, dark toffee, and molasses," it can bring a tear to some gluten-free brewers' eyes. Being an even darker caramel malt, Caramel 240L shares some fermentation characteristics with Caramel 90L and 120L but provides even more color and dark caramel flavors. It can be used in various styles, especially export stouts and imperial stouts. Don't get me wrong, you can achieve a stout using just chocolate millet malt, but I believe the foam color really makes a difference, and the Caramel 240L malt makes sure of a darker foamy head.

MILLET MALT: COLOR OUTSIDE THE LINES

Many people are confused by the ranges given for the colors of these millet malts. When you look at a bag of Grouse's pale millet, or almost any other millet malt for that matter, there are some grains that are often darker than others—this seems to be just a facet of the grain itself.

Rice malt is typically homogeneously colored when it comes out of the kiln, so why not millet? The secret could lie in the size of the millet grain—there are likely grains that are not being fully exposed to the kiln heat and some that are more exposed than others. Another factor could be that Grouse Malt House uses a small-batch artisanal coffee roaster when producing its various roasts. This is one of the main reasons why many of Grouse's medium-level roasts give off coffee flavors. It makes a ton of sense to include a blend of various malts when producing darker styles like stouts so that you can achieve the desired roast and color without losing flavor depth.

BUCKWHEAT

Buckwheat can be found in pale, caramel (around 10°L), and roasted varieties, both malted and unmalted. At time of writing, Grouse Malt House is the main dedicated gluten-free producer of buckwheat malts in the US. With the exception of groats and crystal buckwheat malts, the descriptions are in reference to Grouse products.

Do not be afraid of buckwheat's β-glucan content; lean into it to get some incredible tastes and textures in your finished beers. Buckwheat does have a higher protein content than rice or millet and, as such, can lead to better head retention, but it can also cause troublesome haze. Buckwheat malt is a highly recommended ingredient to aid in the quality of your finished beer, but there is a disclaimer: many brewers have had brew days that ended up being complicated because the grain was treated incorrectly, so make sure that you respect the β-glucans. Complications can involve stuck mashes and long lauter times, so a β-glucan rest during the mash is commonly advised at the homebrew and commercial levels.

β-GLUCAN

β-Glucan is a polysaccharide (a polymer made of sugar units) with a crystalline structure. It is often immune to enzymatic hydrolysis unless treated correctly. Most grains that contain β-glucan also possess β-glucanase enzymes, which tend to denature above 145°F (63°C) so these grains often need a lower rest temperature during the mash to break down these sugars. Barley β-glucans are highly viscous and can cause a number of problems in brewing, notably reduced rates of wort separation and beer filtration and also the formation of hazes, gels, and precipitates (Jin et al., 2004, 231–240).

Despite the industry trend to only use buckwheat up to about 30% of the grain bill, it can in theory be used up to 80%, maybe more, so feel free to experiment. Hesitation on the part of commercial brewers may be because many tasters familiar with barley beers will instantly pick out buckwheat in the aroma as a vegetal, flax seed, castor oil, or even "fishy" smell (although I have never detected a fish note). Start low and gauge your tolerance.

Buckwheat groats (0°L). Buckwheat groats are typically used up to a maximum of 5%–10% of a grain bill. They lend some additional body but not much taste unless you roast them; when roasted, the groats give high levels of nuttiness in both the taste and aroma. There is usually no husk, so drainage will be a consideration and another reason to not use this grain at too high of a rate.

Pale buckwheat malt (1.7–2.8°L). Pale buckwheat malt is a highly useful grain that elicits a warm nuttiness. Tasters will sometimes get a slight vegetal or "umami" note on the nose and palate with a high enough buckwheat content. One thing you will hear over and over when it comes to buckwheat is that it is great for head retention, even when only around 5% of the grain bill. It can fit in just about any flavor profile you are looking to make. There is a lovely thickness that buckwheat brings to any craft beer style that can leave the drinker pleasantly satisfied.

Roasted buckwheat malt (22.7–37.5°L). Roasted buckwheat malt contributes lovely flavors of walnut, maple, and toast. Use this malt in pale ales, amber ales, and various other styles that are complemented by nuttiness.

Crystal buckwheat (10–60°L). Available from the Colorado Malting Company (a non-dedicated malting facility, so cross-contamination concerns apply), crystal buckwheat malts are much harder to source. My favorite hoppy amber (or should I say, chocolate IPA) to date uses crystal buckwheat 30°L. From light caramel (10°L) to toffee and chocolate (60°L), crystal buckwheat is a great addition to your brewing arsenal whenever you can find it.

Caramel buckwheat (10°L). Caramel buckwheat is another innovation out of Grouse Malt House, released in 2021, and likely the missing link in the gluten-free brewing world. Something about the enzymatic processes used in making this grain removes almost all the nuttiness and vegetal taste that buckwheat is known for, leaving behind a malty sweetness that could be the very ingredient that will allow gluten-free beers to compete in barley specific categories and medal regularly.

Roasted unmalted buckwheat. There can sometimes be confusion between roasted buckwheat malt and roasted unmalted buckwheat, so make sure you read the label before buying. Roasted *unmalted* buckwheat can provide wonderful notes of chocolate and cacao nib to a finished beer. If you are targeting buckwheat for its enzymes like β-amylase, unmalted versions will not possess much of any.

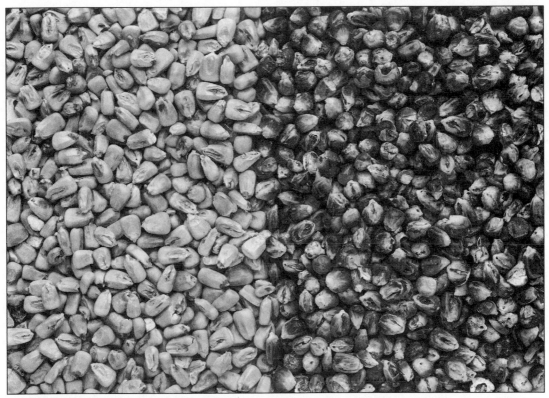

Figure 3.3. Whole, malted corn (maize) contributes additional flavors that flaked corn does not. Depending on the variety, corn can also lend some great color. To date, one of my favorite beers is made with blue corn (right).

CORN (MAIZE)

Although corn (maize) heirloom programs domestically and internationally have brought us a more diverse range of colors in the past century, yellow and blue corn are still the most common varieties you can find out there. Dos Luces Brewery in Denver, CO recently came out with a black chicha in support of the #BlackisBeautiful collaboration project, made from roasted blue corn. I would say that red corn, if that's what you have, is close enough to blue in terms of overall color and taste impact. These new innovations show that corn is still a brewing grain of distinction to be respected and cherished, and not only for its traditional appeal.

As with millet and buckwheat, the descriptions of these malts are in regard to the products from Grouse Malt House.

Organic yellow corn (5°L). By most accounts, yellow corn has a neutral flavor from a malt stand-point, but also a fairly recognizable taste depending on how much of it you use. People love its sharp, crisp, yet often sweet and creamy appeal. But malted, this grain is such an affordable character builder in any beer, even in low quantities (5% or less in the grain bill). When it is malted, its flavors increase, though there seems to be something lost in the flaking process. Whole, malted corn has a superior flavor, and while it still needs to be cooked or used in conjunction with exogenous enzymes, in my experience the flavor is off the charts in a clean fermented beer. A good boil is always recommended.

Organic blue corn (26°L). Blue corn is the base malt for chicherías, that is, breweries that produce chicha (like Dos Luces Brewery), a fermented corn-based beer based on ancient Incan brews. It creates a beer that is ruby, even purple or fuchsia, in color (some haziness can even make it pink). While the color is partly to do with the ending pH of the beer, I have begun to use this malt as a character malt in certain styles to get a red color without any roast taste. In fact, many tasters get a rather unexpected taste from blue corn—there is still a slight creamy, sweet note but also a nutty character that finishes with a slight herbal taste. This grain is screaming out to be put in anything funky, phenolic, fruity, or woodsy; the possibilities are endless as few have even considered using this grain. I have used blue corn at various proportions in the grain bill and with various yeasts, and rarely have the flavors disappointed. One of the hidden gems of the brewing world, this is a grain to have some fun with.

> *One of my favorite recipes involves 50% rice malt with 50% blue corn malt and fermented with Champagne yeast. Very clean and floral, with a slight hint of berry.*

QUINOA

Quinoa (0–9°L) is becoming more readily available as a brewing ingredient; like buckwheat, it is a pseudocereal. Quinoa typically only makes up a low percentage of the grain bill, in part due to its high cost. The grains are small so the flaked form is ideal, unless you are able to puff your quinoa before you brew with it (some grocery aisles may have puffed quinoa for purchase). At time of writing, there was no commercially available malted quinoa product. If you want to brew with malted quinoa, you will probably have to make your own arrangements to have it malted. Very much a superfood, quinoa is laden with amino acids, which promotes high FAN levels and aids with good fermentation. Quinoa's protein content is super helpful in producing lasting foam when you are using highly fermentable yet low-protein grains as your base, like corn, rice, potatoes, or cassava.

When used above 5%–10% of the grain bill you may notice a green pepper taste that quinoa is known for, but typically it lends more of an earthy and sweet nuttiness. This grain is also great for adding a stable haze and increasing head retention, as well as adding viscosity to your beer. A delightful surprise in certain styles, it works quite well in wheat-style clones and Belgian styles alike.

> *Quinoa was not as hard for me to consider as some other gluten-free brewing ingredients. It can get eclectic: fermentables like teff, amaranth, and sunflower seeds are coming onto the market but have not really gained much traction. There are some regional differences in availability that make it hard to recommend these ingredients to every brewer, but they can lead to some awesome flavor profiles. Teff appears to be one that should be approached with care, as it leads to stuck mashes often enough that it's not really worthwhile, but all of these fermentables have featured in some exceptional beers.*

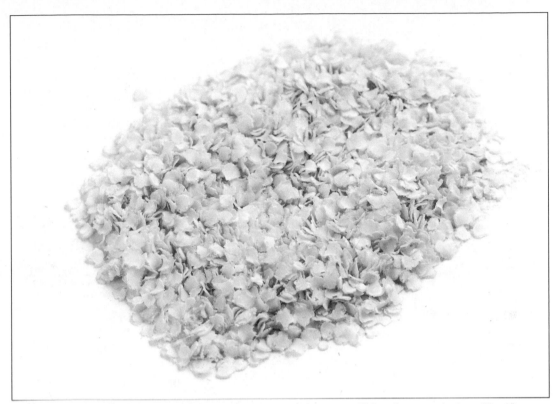

Figure 3.4. A pseudocereal, quinoa is an ancient grain that originated in the Andes. However, this ingredient can modernize traditional flavors and add a more complex spice note to styles like saison. © Getty/rodrigobark

AMARANTH

Amaranth (1°L) lends a malty, nutty note that can go great with various beer styles. You will have to malt it yourself, however, if you would like to have the full experience, as it is not currently available from any large malt houses. You will also need to roast it yourself, so some do-it-yourself grit is needed if you are to get the most out of this grain in brewing.

SUNFLOWER SEEDS

Sunflower seeds (0°L) are an adjunct highly recommended for haze-heads as they make a consistently hazy beer. The nuttiness from this ingredient is a little bit overpowering at times; use restraint with this adjunct as it can throw you out of style. It is great for any experimental style, however, and I could see it doing well in milkshake IPAs specifically (as well as other hop-dominant styles). Currently, there is no commercially available sunflower seed malt made in a dedicated gluten-free malthouse, so cross contamination may be a concern if purchasing malted seeds in the US.

UNUSUAL ADJUNCTS

Adjuncts like unmalted chestnuts, lentils, and alder catkins are all ingredients that can lend a malty note to a gluten-free beer. They are especially useful if you are brewing on a budget. For US brewers, items like chestnuts and alder catkins may be easier to find in certain states than others. Depending on how you use them, you could pull some outside-of-style flavors in your finished product, so carefully dialing in quantities is important. Remember that truly world-class beer is produced by wort, yeast stewardship, and packaging procedures, and not necessarily what is used in making it.

After I made a comment on a HomebrewTalk.com article about brewing with non-traditional ingredients, a brewer in the northern Midwest contacted me directly and mentioned that they forage and use alder catkins to create malty flavors when they cannot source gluten-free malts and adjuncts reliably. Although I have not personally tried alder catkins in practice, they are worth considering if sourcing gluten-free ingredients that provide malty flavors is difficult where you are in the world.

Table 3.1. Commonly used gluten-free malts and adjuncts with suggested mash treatments and expected extract yields

Grain (Malted)	α-Amylase for Self-Conversion	β-Amylase for Self-Conversion	Limit Dextrinase for Self-Conversion	Exogenous Enzymes Needed?	High-Temp. Step Needed? (Above 170°F/76°C)	Protein or β-Glucan Treatment?	Expected PPG (l°/kg)
Sorghum	Yes	No	No	Yes	Yes	No	33 (275)
Rice	No	No	No	Yes	Yes	No	31 (259)
Millet	Yes	Partial	Yes	Dependent on brewhouse capabilities	Yes	No	29 (242)
Corn (maize)	No	No	No	Yes	Yes	No	29 (242)
Oats	Yes	Yes	Yes	No	No	Yes	25 (209)
Teff	No	Yes	No	Yes	Yes	Yes	25 (209)

Pseudocereal (Malted)	α-Amylase for Self-Conversion	β-Amylase for Self-Conversion	Limit Dextrinase for Self-Conversion	Exogenous Enzymes Needed?	High-Temp. Step Needed? (Above 170°F/76°C)	Protein or β-Glucan Treatment?	Expected PPG (l°/kg)
Quinoa*	Unknown	Unknown	Unknown	Yes	Yes	Yes	31 (259)
Buckwheat	No	Yes	No	Yes	Yes	Yes	28 (234)
Amaranth*	Unknown	Unknown	Unknown	Yes	Yes	Yes	28 (234)

Table 3.1 continued on next page »

Table 3.1. (cont.)

Adjuncts (Whole)	α-Amylase for Self-Conversion	β-Amylase for Self-Conversion	Limit Dextrinase for Self-Conversion	Exogenous Enzymes Needed?	High-Temp. Step Needed? (Above 170°F/76°C)	Protein or β-Glucan Treatment?	Expected PPG (l°/kg)
Chestnuts	No	No	No	Yes	No	No	20 (167)
Tapioca/cassava starch	No	No	No	Yes	Yes	No	11.5 (96)
Sunflower seed (malted)	No	No	No	Yes	No	Yes	4 (33)
Lentils	No	No	No	Yes	Yes	Yes	0 (0)
Sweet potato (whole)	Yes	Yes	No	No	Yes	No	8 (67)
Sweet potato (flaked)	No	No	No	Yes	Yes	No	35 (292)
White potato (whole)	No	No	No	Yes	Yes	No	8 (67)
White potato (flaked)	No	No	No	Yes	Yes	No	35 (292)
Beet (whole)	No	No	No	Yes	Yes	No	2 (17)

Notes: Endogenous enzymes necessary for self-conversion (α-amylase, β-amylase, and limit dextrinase) are listed. For most, exogenous enzymes are necessary for the mash to produce a fermentable wort. Some grains and adjuncts require a high-temperature step to allow conversion to take place, and some require a protein or β-glucan treatment.
* Not available as commercially malted products at time of publication. Requires at-home malting.

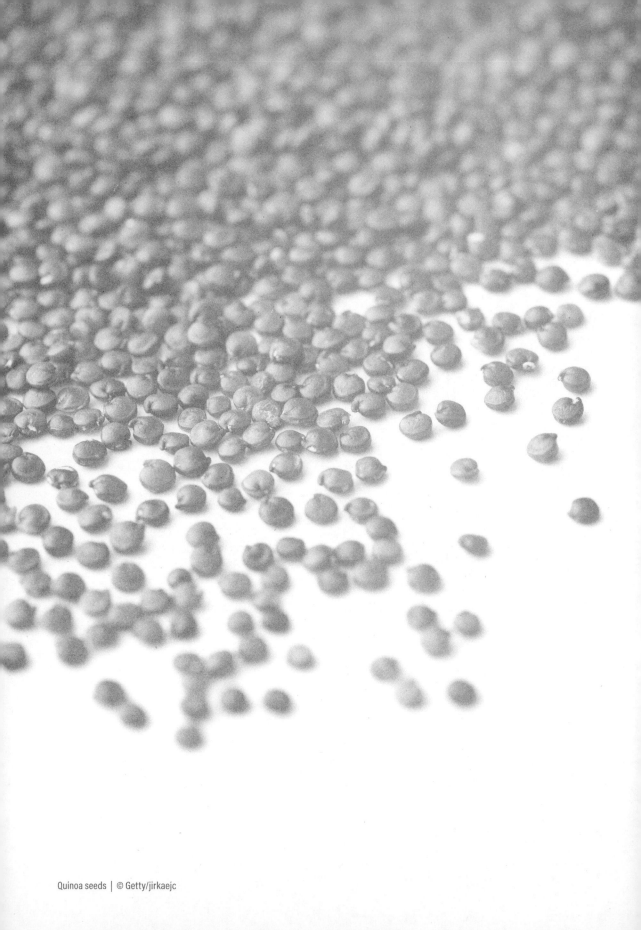

Quinoa seeds | © Getty/jirkaejc

4

Recipe Formulation

You could write volumes on just recipe formulation in gluten-free brewing, because there are so many ingredients and flavors on the table. In this chapter, we will focus on brewing to style with gluten-free grains in traditional competition categories. There are various homebrew and commercial style guidelines that influenced this chapter, but I have not adhered to any particular set of competition rules as they change and evolve every year. Additionally, there are some sections where enzymes and mash techniques are referenced. Please refer to chapter 5, where we go more in depth into various techniques a gluten-free brewer can use to achieve various styles, which is somewhat more nuanced than the techniques a barley brewer typically uses.

ENTERING COMPETITIONS WITH THE INTENT TO WIN

In theory, any category is up for entry when you are brewing gluten free, whether you have got your eyes on the podium or just looking for feedback. Do not get me wrong, the gluten-free category is the obvious place for a gluten-free beer as no other barley or wheat-based beer can compete in that category, but in practice there is no barrier of entry to other categories for the gluten-free brewer. When you are setting your sights on traditional flavors, it is important to understand where you are coming close and where your grain selection, packaging issues, or a plethora of other elements are pushing your beer away from the style you are emulating. Judges' gentle nudges, malt selection advice (which can be translated by studying the flavors that the suggested malt provides and finding a close gluten-free analog), or fermentation notes can help you down the road in future competitions.

> *When entering into any beer competition, the focus should always be to submit to the category that truly represents the beer you brewed, not necessarily the beer you set out to brew. This is as true for brewers of gluten-free beer as it is for any other brewer.*

The wort you create and your yeast stewardship are crucial to making great beer. Gluten-free beer can have some of the same issues that barley-based beer can have, often for the same reasons, but there may be a few issues unique to some of the ingredients used in gluten-free brewing. Conversely, gluten-free grains are sometimes immune to certain issues found with conventional brewing grains, although this field of study is only just beginning.

RECIPE BASICS

There are some broad issues to consider before you start putting together a specific recipe. Gluten-free grains may behave differently to barley and wheat when mashing, so if you are coming from a background of brewing with conventional grains you may need to slightly adjust some of your best practices when it comes to making gluten-free beer. That said, all hops are still on the table, and there is a plethora of dry yeasts, and the occasional liquid yeast, that are available and safe for gluten-free beers, as we spoke about in chapter 2 (p. 25).

Using tools like BrewersFriend and BeerSmith can save you time and are recommended when attempting to clone certain beers or create entirely new ones. In fact, additions to these platforms by members of the gluten-free community have made it easier than ever to create a gluten-free recipe, as almost the whole catalog of malts and grains available from Grouse and Eckert malthouses have already been loaded into these programs by gluten-free brewers. BeerSmith even offers stats that will help you optimize calculations and steps specific to certain mash techniques.[1] These tools also allow you to enter your own custom grains, adjuncts, and relevant stats (like expected extract potential and color values) if you are using ingredients the tool does not possess. Additionally, brewing groups like the Zero Tolerance Gluten Free Homebrew Club have great "getting started" recipes, and members are constantly posting beers, recipes, and tasting notes.

> *I have spent countless hours on various forums but, in the end, all I learned was that I was powerful thirsty after all that reading. If you start feeling "analysis paralysis," just grab some sorghum syrup (or whatever gluten-free syrup is easiest to source), hops, and yeast at your local homebrew supply store and at least get started so you have something to drink while you are doing research.*

WATER

Water is the most important element of any beer, period. John Palmer and Colin Kaminski (2012) wrote at length on this topic in their book *Water*, and I highly recommend adding this book to your reading list.

To start, knowing the profile of your water source can make a huge difference. Gluten-free grains benefit from brewing salts. Adding salts like calcium chloride and calcium sulfate (gypsum) are great if you are building your water from the "blank slate" of reverse osmosis-treated water, specifically because they aid in mash pH stability, which is vital for specific enzymes. Mash pH can have a massive impact on sugar extraction as well as the overall flavor of the

---

[1] An example of this is doing a falling temperature step mash (refer to chapter 5). With this technique, you might be starting with a smaller volume of higher temperature mash liquid so that you can gelatinize certain grains. BeerSmith can help you understand how adding additional grain and water will help you achieve a specific second temperature rest by doing the calculations for you.

final beer. Because many gluten-free grains tend to create a more alkaline mash and many such grains gelatinize at higher temperatures than barley, tannin extraction can be an issue throughout the mash process. The best practice for lowering your all-grain mash pH is to use organic acids, like citric acid, lactic acid, or phosphoric acid, to achieve the correct conditions for your enzymes (both endogenous and exogenous). The pros know that when you get your mash pH right tannic extraction is not a concern—mash water temperatures that exceed traditional lautering/sparging temperatures is then mainly a concern for enzymatic activities or for special processes like a ferulic acid rest.

Yeast naturally lowers the pH of beer during fermentation, so keeping the mash pH between 5.2 and 5.6 will help your beers finish at a pH of 4.2 to 4.6. Given that many gluten-free grains will not buffer mash pH in the same way as conventional brewing grains, and the fact that the use of exogenous enzymes often necessitates pushing mash pH slightly higher than you might find in a conventional barley mash, it is crucial for gluten-free brewers to pay close attention to their mash pH. Dialing in your starting pH will help avoid off-flavors due to poor yeast health from the yeast being outside of its optimal pH. Yeast health is the main concern here: lower fermentation pH levels can lead to certain off-flavors, and fermentation pH levels above 5.9 can also lead to off-flavors. The nature of the off-flavors differs depending on whether the pH was too high or too low. For example, a low pH can result in a slightly sharp beer that may be rescuable, whereas a high pH can result in astringency and an unstable, starchy, hazy beer.

Various mash techniques can successfully produce good gluten-free beers, and chapter 5 will be dedicated to exploring several of these techniques.

MALT

The reason for using malt in beer is that it contains nutrients that yeast can use, which greatly impacts the final taste of the beer. The absence of these nutrients in some syrups or unmalted grains will negatively impact fermentation, which can contribute to off-flavors. Thus, adding yeast nutrient is typically a necessary step when using these ingredients.

For gluten-free malts, the situation is better nutrient-wise. Although millet malt is not really modified to the degree that barley and wheat malts are, it still contains a great deal of yeast food. However, bear in mind that millet will need a gelatinization rest temperature that is outside of the ideal temperature ranges for most enzymes involved in the "classic" mash rests. Nevertheless, millet is a great source of nutrients like calcium, copper, iron, magnesium, phosphorus, potassium, and selenium as well as essential vitamins like folate (B_9), pantothenic acid (B_5), niacin (B_3), riboflavin (B_2), pyridoxine (B_6), and vitamins C, E, and K. These nutrients are also present in broadly similar amounts in buckwheat, rice, sorghum, and quinoa. When used in the right way, oftentimes paired together, these gluten-free cereals and pseudocereals are certainly capable of supporting healthy fermentations and creating medal-worthy beers. In fact, many barley brewers have been incorporating them into recipes, and beer tasters have not been able to spot flaws when these grains are used.[2]

Rice does make a lot of sense when you consider its clean flavor, despite there being some risks of off-flavors if proper yeast health is not maintained. However, I recommend using malts with a higher friability than rice when you are first starting out with gluten-free brewing. Millet tops the list of base malts suitable for a beginner to all-grain gluten-free brewing. Sorghum and oat malts, while recently becoming easier to source, are at present not as widely available as millet malt. Sorghum and oat malts also need special mash regimes and nutrient additions to get good extraction and healthy yeast fermentations; and don't forget that oats elicit an autoimmune reaction in around 20% of people with celiac disease. Buckwheat, corn, and quinoa are great additions, but their more noticeable flavor contributions (see chapter 3) mean they are better used in lower quantities rather than making up the majority of the base malt.

[2] Andy Carter and SoCAl Cerveceros, "ExBEERiment: Caramel Malt: Barley vs. Millet in an American Amber Ale," *Brülosophy*, 18 December, 2021, https://brulosophy.com/2021/12/20/exbeeriment-caramel-malt-barley-vs-millet-in-an-american-amber-ale/.

MILLING

Gluten-free grains are smaller than their gluten-containing relatives, and that poses its own problems with both milling and the use of false bottoms in the mash tun. Milling helps with starch extraction and also drainage; a coarser grind tends to allow for easier lautering or sparging. Coarser grinds result in less efficiency, requiring the use of more malt to achieve target gravity (a not insignificant cost concern with gluten-free malts).

As you may expect, mill gap settings will need to be adjusted depending on the gluten-free grains that you are using. For malted or unmalted whole grain millet, amaranth, corn, sorghum, and buckwheat a gap setting of 0.55–0.70 mm is preferred. For malted whole grain rice and oats, however, a 0.90–0.95 mm gap setting is better. Smaller grains like quinoa and teff, because they are so tiny, work better with mill gap settings of 0.50 mm and below. With the correct milling, there is often no need for rice hulls since the grains themselves should set up the correct drainage.

For homebrewers, there are plenty of mill types to choose from in this day and age. From dedicated roller mills available from various purveyors, to Corona® Mills, KitchenAid® attachments, spice grinders, triple-blade Ninja® blenders, and all the way to the time-tested stone grinding by hand, there are plenty of ways to go about crushing your grains. From personal experience, I have found that Ninja blenders do a great job, especially with rice, which has a much denser endosperm than millet. Millet would only need about 10–15 seconds of pulsing before being the right consistency, whereas rice often took 45–60 seconds before being the right consistency. After years of using the household Ninja blender, my loving wife gifted me a grain mill that I could use with her KitchenAid, and, although it is a unitask device, it has been a wonderful addition to my home brewhouse.

HOPPING GLUTEN-FREE BEER

Hopping regimes for gluten-free beers will tend to be the same as those for barley-based brews. Base your dosage on the wort gravity as you would normally. However, the frequently increased fermentability of worts in gluten-free brewing is something to consider, as you can accidentally increase the perceived bitterness of your beer if it overattenuates (e.g., you may create a de facto triple IPA if you ferment all the sugars out of your gluten-free double IPA). So, for hopping, choosing the right type of mash for your beer is just as important as the hop varieties you select.

BEER STYLE CONSIDERATIONS

Using millet, rice, buckwheat, quinoa, sorghum, and oats (plus some adjuncts) as our main focus for recipe development, let us build recipes from the guidelines and flavor profiles we learned about in chapters 2 and 3. With so many competition-defined beer styles out there, it was difficult to narrow down the selection for this part. The style considerations that follow are inspired by beers currently available commercially from gluten-free breweries, as well as by recipes that were sent in from brewers for use in chapters 6–10. Additionally, some styles were chosen to show the contrast between guidelines of similar beer styles that, at the competition level, are treated as very distinct beers and judged strictly; think of, for example, different types of wheat beers, different types of lagers, or even when considering the more subtle distinctions of dry Irish stout compared with porter. I've said it before: Listen to your beer. What I mean by this is that, although some style guidelines can be blurry, the guidelines are there for a reason. Your best laid brewing plans may still result in a different beer style, and it is your job as the brewer to correctly categorize your beer or it's just not going to go the distance. And that's OK if it doesn't exactly land, stylistically speaking, where you intended—beer speaks in many ways, you just have to have your senses tuned in to what it's saying.

BASE MALT VERSUS CHARACTER MALT

What is a base malt and what is a character malt? Honestly, in gluten-free brewing, it can be tough to tell sometimes. The main difficulty in defining a base malt in gluten-free brewing is that, since exogenous enzymes are so commonly used, you do not need a millet malt or a sorghum malt for diastatic power (and rice malts have no diastatic power at all). Even though they lend wonderful flavors, there isn't a preset "base" quantity of these malts that is assigned when setting out to brew gluten free.

What this means in practice is that you could make a beer from 100% Goldfinch Millet Malt, or 100% amber rice malt. The resulting beers would certainly have ample flavor, but may lack the depth you are going for, which is one of the main reasons I will suggest using particular combinations of "base" malts to achieve certain styles. Some malts contribute certain flavors that obviously will increase when used in larger doses, and this is often a reason your gluten-free version of a beer may be deemed "out of style" depending on what you set out to brew. This may take some getting used to when you start brewing gluten free, but at least dialing in recipes is usually a pretty tasty learning experience.

WHEAT BEERS

German-style hefeweizen. Hefeweizen is a style that balances fruity and phenolic ("banana clove") with a noticeably full mouthfeel due to proteins and some yeast in suspension. A grain bill involving a blend of millet, rice, and lentils would achieve this balance easily. Some small quantities of flaked quinoa, unmalted raw oats, or raw or malted corn (maize) are a great idea to help achieve the correct flavor and mouthfeel, but the focus should be on malty, bready, and fruity-spice flavor profiles. Buckwheat and quinoa can often put off more green pepper and pink peppercorn, which is great in a witbier but is not to style for a hefeweizen. Both rice and corn possess high levels of ferulic acid in their bran and kernel, respectively (Boz 2015, 2), and those clove and banana flavors may be elevated further by stressing the yeast during fermentation. This can be done by taking steps to add additional glucose to the wort (rice and corn provide this quite easily), taking steps to solubilize the intrinsic ferulic acid during the mash (with specific enzymes or rest temperatures), or by constantly changing the temperature between lower and higher ranges of the yeast's tolerance during primary fermentation.

Rising step mashes are commonly used when brewing German-style hefeweizens, although a ferulic acid rest at around 108°F (42°C) is used specifically to hydrolyze the insoluble ferulic acid found in wheat bran. There seems to be some credence to applying this principle when brewing gluten free, but mash process is honestly more determined by brewhouse limitations and the exogenous enzymes you are using, as we will see in chapter 5. Therefore, adding the right ingredients with the correct flavor precursors should be the focus in this style of beer. That is why both rice and corn are advisable when approaching this style in gluten-free form, since they have the most readily available ferulic acid levels and will bring you closer to style. The main reason for the rising step mash in gluten-free brewing is for the protein and β-glucan rests that will benefit a high-adjunct style like this, although these rests are not always necessary depending on the enzymes used.

Commercial examples: Aurochs Hefe (Aurochs Brewing Co.)

Belgian-style witbier. Belgian witbier is typically straw to yellow in color, hazy, with mild spice, fruit (often citrus), and yeast flavors present. The best base malts for a gluten-free Belgian-style witbier are millet and buckwheat, but various additional grains can be considered. Sorghum malt could be a good base for the overall flavor, at least 50% of the fermentables; however, you will need to add haze-stabilizing adjuncts in a sorghum-heavy grain bill. Sorghum syrup is a great choice since it can add a certain citrus bitterness by itself, which helps you lean into the flavors this style in known for.

I also recommend some unmalted grains like millet seed or buckwheat groats to achieve the flavor profiles you're looking for. For a creamy note, some blue corn is also advisable, and can help add different types of spice notes as well as some color. If safe for you, rolled oats are also a good idea for creaminess and haze stability; you may achieve the similar results with oat malt, but rolled oats are better here. Rice, even with the potential for off-flavors (specifically rice's potential for wintergreen), if present in small quantities could be admissible in a style like this as well.

Starch left in suspension is a good thing in this style. There are many ways to devise an appropriate mash strategy for this when brewing gluten free. Since gluten-free brewing is often, by nature, "high-adjunct" brewing, you are already most of the way there in terms of creating a starchy (unconverted) wort. So think of this more from an unmalted standpoint. In theory, you could also just decrease the amount of enzymes used to get an appropriate amount of leftover starch, rather than balancing the grain bill like you would with a barley or wheat-based mash. You could also not use enzymes at all (see chapter 5 for the decantation method).

Orange peel and spices (namely, coriander) are typically featured in witbiers but these flavors also arise from a properly selected Belgian yeast, or you can in theory achieve some of those same flavors with hops (late boil hops could give a modern take on this historic style). You could even envision it as a toned-down hazy IPA recipe, with much less hopping during fermentation but similar kettle and whirlpool hopping techniques—this can also add to haze stability; then ferment with a dry witbier yeast and you can get pretty close to style.

The Belgian witbier style has a fair amount of leeway, and citrus and spice are something that gluten-free grains do really well, even if you do not add any spices during the brewing or fermentation process. Through my years of brewing, this is my favorite style to come back to because I rarely make the same wit twice.

Commercial examples: Shrouded Summit (Ghostfish Brewing Company), BuckWit Belgian (Holidaily Brewing Co.), Glutenberg White (Glutenberg)

COMPARING GOSE AND BERLINER WEISSE

The two German styles, Gose and Berliner Weisse, have a lot in common. The classic styles both typically contain wheat, are tart to sour, and are cloudy, highly attenuated beers. But they are distinct styles and it is important to know how they differ.

Gose styles. Gose differs from its fellow tart East German counterpart due to it possessing salt as well as coriander in the recipe. These recipe components can be found in historical Gose, Leipzig Gose, and contemporary Gose recipes.

There are some key distinctions to be made within these Gose variations. If you plan to add a fruit element (even the peels), you will not want to enter into the Leipzig or historical Gose categories because fruit additions are not to style here. When approaching this as a gluten-free brewer, you might also need to be selective with malt choice depending on which category you plan to enter. For example, sorghum is likely not a good choice in Leipzig Gose, but would be a great choice in contemporary or historical Gose due to the fruity notes that sorghum contributes, and that the latter beers are more known for. Oats are commonly noted in Gose styles, so rolled or malted is a good choice and are to style, whether brewing Leipzig, historical, or contemporary Gose. Additionally, malts like pale buckwheat and flaked quinoa could be great choices as well if you are using a yeast that lends spicy phenols.

One additional element is color: contemporary Gose versions with added fruit will likely take on the color of the added fruit, but a Leipzig Gose is noted for its straw to amber color. Due to the cloudiness of classic Gose, a brewer should select neutral flavored character malts, like Munich millet malt (from Grouse) or a lighter biscuit rice malt (Eckert), as malt sweetness should be low if perceivable at all in this style. To achieve an amber color you could consider other malts, but you will likely want to use them at or below the 5% threshold to avoid contributing too many flavors that will throw you out of style.

Commercial examples: Gosefish (Ghostfish Brewing Company), Glutenberg Gose (Glutenberg), Citrus Gose (Holidaily Brewing Co.), New Grist Gose-Style with Lime (Lakefront Brewery), Hibiscus Lime Gose (Moonshrimp Brewing), Margarita Sour (Two Bays Brewing Co.)

Berliner weisse. Berliner weiss is a wheat beer, which means that it will typically feature up to 50% wheat malt. As such, many of the same recommendations from the discussion on German-style hefeweizen (p. 63) could be applied in this category. Where Berliner weisse differs is in the yeast and bacteria that ferment the wort, creating the tart, fruity, and phenolic profile the style is known for. While Berliner weisse is commonly packaged with fruit, any such examples are better served in the specialty Berliner weisse category if you're going to competition.

Commercial examples: Sour Berliner Weiss (Bierly Brewing)

PUMPKIN/SQUASH SPICE BEER

Many beer styles can be altered with adjuncts and spices, but pumpkin spice beers are perhaps the epitome of this. In competitions, this can be a tough category to earn a medal in because it is highly competitive, with many entrants and such a wide variety of styles. Top ingredients to consider are malted sorghum, malted buckwheat, flaked quinoa, sweet potato, cassava, and malted rice; but you can look to just about anything you have on hand, since the top-placing beers in this category can differ widely and entrants are often required to write in the specialty ingredients used or the context of these ingredients and how they relate to the beer style presented. Squash can be featured in the mash, kettle, or primary *or* secondary fermentation, so the possibilities there are endless. Traditional pumpkin spice involves cinnamon, allspice, clove, and nutmeg, but you can also consider various other spices, such as a wit-pumpkin (coriander), vanilla pumpkin robust porter, or coffee pumpkin pastry stout. Cardamom also works well in this style. As long as you represent the base style well, you will have a shot with the judges. Molasses is another adjunct that comes to mind for squash and spice beer but avoid using it above 10% of the recipe to keep metallic tastes low, especially if you plan to use sorghum syrup as your base fermentable, which itself can cause an often referenced "twang" for the taster.

A dextrinous wort is best practice with gluten-free spice beer due to the body you will lose if you use ingredients like rice, sweet potato, cassava, and sorghum. Adjuncts that add body, like buckwheat and quinoa, are also great considerations.

Commercial examples: Old Man Sage (MoonShrimp Brewing), Patchy Waters Pumpkin Ale (Holidaily Brewing Co.), Lunar Harvest (Ghostfish Brewing Company), Pumpkin Belgian Ale (Bierly Brewing), Glutenator (Epic Brewing)

AMERICAN-STYLE BLONDE ALE

An American-style blonde ale is an all-day-drinking kind of beer. Light straw to gold and low in alcohol, with a clear aspect, malty/cereal taste, and low hop perception. Millet, rice, corn, and oats—even sweet potato and sorghum—make sense when making a gluten-free blonde ale. Although GABF guidelines list the finishing gravity as 1.008 for blonde ales, 1.002–1.006 FG is not uncommon in gluten-free versions, so an unmalted grain like millet or flaked quinoa or a malted pseudocereal like buckwheat is recommended in order to retain mouthfeel but not interfere with the clean taste. This style calls for clarity, so cold conditioning is ideal, as well as using highly flocculent yeast and filtering or using a clarifying agent. Fruity hops pair well late in the boil, but earthy, noble hops are just as great. A soft water profile can make a huge difference in this style, as it will better accentuate the malts used.

Commercial examples: Meteor Shower (Ghostfish Brewing Company), Blonde (Evasion Brewing), Aurochs Blonde Ale (Aurochs Brewing Co.), Favorite Blonde (Holidaily Brewing Co.), Two Goldens (Rolling Mills Brewing Company), Glutenberg Blonde (Glutenberg).

AMERICAN CREAM ALE

Unlike with American blonde ale, fruity tastes and aromas are commonly not a feature of cream ale. This style should be crisp with a subtle to medium malt sweetness; base malts like millet and rice, with character ingredients like Goldfinch Millet Malt, Cara Millet malt, malted corn (blue and yellow), and rolled oats all make sense. Though the name seems to suggest a "creamy" mouthfeel, the target for this style is more of a velvety smoothness. While grains like corn and oats can contribute a creamy mouthfeel, that is not necessary to style but can be helpful tools in the gluten-free brewer's arsenal. That said, cream ale can be approached from a few different angles as this style can feature ale or lager yeast, or a combination of the two. Cream ales are also known for being rather dry, just like blonde ale, and often the line between these styles is blurry.

As with lagers or Kölsch, cream ale calls for a deft, balanced hand when using malts and hops, with American "noble" hops dominating this category.

Commercial examples: Event Horizon Blonde[3] (Divine Science Brewing), Cream Ale (Mutantis)

PALE ALE (BRITISH AND AMERICAN)

Some interpretations of pale ale are not actually that pale since they traditionally feature high quantities of Maris Otter in the British versions and, more commonly in American versions, crystal barley malts, so the colors can range from gold to copper. With herbal or earthy hop character in British styles, and citrus and stone or tropical fruit hop character in American styles, malt takes a little bit more of a backseat in pale ale, but balance is still important for both. A medium fruit character from the yeast and hops with medium body is in style on either side of the pond.

For gluten-free pale ales, using high-protein malts like buckwheat, quinoa, and oats makes sense, with careful attention paid to developing a clean malt profile, as spice and phenols are not to style in pale ale categories. Grouse Malt House's caramel buckwheat and Cara Millet, and even their Dutch Roast, Red Wing, darker caramel, and Roasted Goldfinch millet malts, make sense for creating balance when used in the right quantities. One recommendation is a light touch of some crystal or amber rice malt from Eckert Malting and Brewing to nail the copper tone of this style.

Since pale ales are more hop forward, sorghum syrup or sorghum malt makes sense for the fruitiness sorghum contributes on its own and, possibly when paired with high-protein ingredients like buckwheat or lentils, will achieve the appropriate body and lasting head retention.

There is such a range of color in pale ales that you can go in many different directions with your malt bill or hop selection. I truly love this style, as someone who grew up in Northern California, home of probably the widest known American pale ale in the world (and was my first experience of craft beer).

Commercial examples: Vanishing Point (Ghostfish Brewing Company), Inclusion (Ground Breaker Brewing), Pale Ale (Buck Wild Brewing), Pale Ale (New Planet Beer), Anti-Federalist Pale Ale (Rolling Mills Brewing Company), Pale Ale (Two Bays Brewing Co.)

PALE ALE: A QUICK COMPARISON OF BRITISH AND AMERICAN STYLES

British and American pale ales are two highly popular styles with their own rich histories. While one is inspired by the other, there are some noticeable differences to the point that it is necessary to mention the country of origin when talking about pale ales.

American versions tend to have more of a caramel note in the aroma and taste. While American pale ales are frequently lighter in aspect than their cousins across the Atlantic, a deeper caramel color is not inappropriate in American styles. Hop perception is similar, but many of the hop flavor contributions differ. For example, although some herbal flavors and aromas are to style, citrus and stone fruit make more sense in American versions and can be added more of liberally than in their UK counterparts. Pale ales are typically dry hopped, but American versions are typically more heavy-handed in this regard.

---

[3] At Divine Science, our Event Horizon is marketed as a blonde ale, but I believe it really is more of a cream ale. The line can be blurry sometimes as hop perception is typically low in both styles.

AMERICAN-STYLE IPA

When aiming for an American IPA, what else is there to say besides go big, bold, and all sorts of hoppy. This is a style that is so free-form it is basically begging gluten-free brewers to enter. In fact, you can approach this style with almost any grain bill. Some gluten-free versions of this style include all of the following ingredients: sorghum, millet, rice, corn, buckwheat, beet sugar, and cane sugar. Increase the mineral content of your water to show off the hops, or lower the mineral levels to show off the malt. Tastes change every year and, yes, the IBU wars of old have all but died out, but your IPA *has* to be hop forward. For gluten-free IPAs you are bringing to competitions, the biggest thing to watch for is that versions brewed with darker malts, non-traditional ale yeasts, fruits, spices, or other flavorings are often categorized as "experimental" instead (e.g., in the GABF®).

Commercial examples: Third Contact IPA (Divine Science Brewing), West-Coast IPA (Buck Wild Brewing), #PacificNorthBlessed (Evasion Brewing), Lucky IPA (Bierly Brewing), IPA No. 5 (Ground Breaker Brewing), Kick Step IPA (Ghostfish Brewing Company), Fat Randy's IPA (Holidaily Brewing Co.), Glutenberg IPA (Glutenberg)

> The list of commercial examples for American IPAs could include a whole lot more, as every brewery making gluten-free beer touts an IPA. There are some experimental IPAs available, like Grapefruit IPA (Ghostfish) and Hophoria (Evasion), and Amber IPA (Bierly); there are also a few Double IPAs, like Hoptensity (Evasion), Peak Buster (Ghostfish), and Double IPA (Glutenberg).

JUICY, OR HAZY, IPA

A juicy, or hazy, IPA is a cloudy aroma bomb with a silky, full mouthfeel. The "juiciness" is from heavy hop use, particularly mid-fermentation dry hopping that allows for biotransformation (conversion by yeast) of hop components into a stable haze with juicy and fruity aromas. While any base malt can be considered, there are specific additional steps that will need to be taken to ensure the correct mouthfeel. Adjuncts like lactose or maltodextrin can contribute additional body and a fuller mouthfeel as well as residual sweetness to balance the hop perception.

For gluten-free versions, just about any base malt (e.g., millet, rice, or sorghum) can be paired with ingredients like unmalted or malted oats and other high-protein adjuncts (e.g., quinoa, buckwheat, and lentils) for creating haze, as the adjunct proteins help stabilize the products of biotransformation. Juicy/hazy IPAs are not known for being too bitter, but some degree of piney and other traditional hop flavors are allowed. Many see this style as an opportunity to create regional variations, like a New England IPA (all fruit and juice) versus a West Coast Hazy (all pine and dank), and style category updates like this could be just around the corner.

Commercial examples: Big Henry Hazy IPA (Holidaily Brewing Co.), Aurochs Hazy IPA (Aurochs Brewing Co.), It Came From The Haze (Ghostfish Brewing's hazy IPA series), Particle Haze (Divine Science Brewing), Double Haze and Huge Monster Hazy (Ground Breaker Brewing), Sonic Bloom (Otherwise Brewing), Hazy IPA (Buck Wild Brewing)

AMERICAN AMBER AND RED ALES

American amber and red ales are known for malt sweetness and some caramel; roast and fruity notes are usually not prominent in this style. Hopping rates can differ quite widely in this style, and various hopping techniques can be used. Go too hoppy, however, and you may want to consider a different category, as too much bitterness would not be to either style.

Previous to Grouse's and Eckert's crystal and caramel malt programs (see chapter 3 for examples), a gluten-free brewer would need to use colored syrups, but with the character malts now available the possibilities are almost endless. In theory, Grouse's caramel millet malts all the way up to Caramel 240L, and Eckert's crystal, amber, and James' Brown Rice malts all make sense when approaching this style. Even still, looking at new millet malts from Grouse's "high dry" program like the dark Munich, roasted Vienna, and Griffin Millet malts, you could in theory approach amber or red ale recipes with these malts as your base grain (up to 60% of the grain bill), and then add caramel buckwheat or flaked quinoa in smaller quantities for additional mouthfeel and texture.

Commercial examples: Red Ale (Glutenberg), Irish Red (Bierly Brewing), Beulah Red (Holidaily Brewing Co.), Amber Ale (Buck Wild Brewing), Discovery Amber Ale (Green's)

DARK MILD

Ahh yes, dark mild, a highly drinkable session dark ale. Dark milds are characterized by restraint and clean fermentation, with some fruity aromas, delivering caramel, licorice, and roast all in balance. Many base malts could be considered, but the focus should be on clean flavors with malty and bready notes; good candidates include pale millet malt, pale rice malt, or even Vienna and Munich millet malts.

Eckert Malting and Brewing's James' Brown Rice malt and darker millet malts from Grouse—its caramel, Dutch Roast, Cara Millet, and Red Wing malts—immediately come to mind when considering character malts to employ for a dark mild. You can include Eckert's Pitch Black rice malt up to 0.5% of the grain bill, which will help you will extract incredible color and some awesome flavors without turning the beer into a stout. Gluten-free versions brewed to style here can be pretty dry, despite having a malt-forward taste, due to gluten-free grains finishing a little drier. These beers routinely range down to 3% ABV, great for beginning all-grain gluten-free brewers, since you do not have to invest in a lot of grain to make this style. If a partial mash is more your speed, and since fruit is one of the flavor goals with this style, using a syrup like unmalted sorghum syrup as a base malt can often lend those flavor notes to the final beer, as long as the you steep darker grains in a partial mash. You would of course need to employ character malts to get the correct flavors in this style, but just about any clean-tasting base is a great idea here.

Commercial example: Dark Ale (Ground Breaker Brewing)

SCOTTISH-STYLE EXPORT ALE

Scottish-style export ale should be medium amber to dark chestnut brown with sweet malt and caramel flavors. Since this is a medium bodied, caramel-forward beer, character malts and grains like Grouse's caramel millet, gluten-free malted oats, and caramel buckwheat, as well as Eckert's crystal rice, are all great choices due to their clean sweetness. All-grain is going to be a much better route to the podium in this category. Grouse's Caramel 90L as well as the newer darker malts (e.g., Griffin Millet malt and darker Munich millet from the "high dry" program) make sense, but going too dark could push you into a different style. As with the ale wine category that follows, this style does also benefit from a longer boil; in theory, you don't always need dark gluten-free malts when approaching this style, as you can achieve a ruddy color or tint to the finished beer with kettle caramelization from a longer boil. Employing a method like this may also help achieve traditional flavors faster than relying on syrups to achieve the correct color, as the wrong flavors (fruit, specifically) could negatively impact a judge's opinion of the resulting beer.

STRONG ALE AND ALE WINE (OR "BARLEY" WINE)

Caramelly, malty, boozy, and oftentimes sticky in stronger versions—strong ales and barley wines are the beers you typically open when you have at least one other drinking buddy to help you drink them. For the most part, the only grains I might suggest staying away from are the darkest roasts, since those could unwittingly throw you into the imperial stout or baltic porter categories. Otherwise, balancing various base malts like pale millet, Vienna or Munich millet malts, pale or biscuit rice malts, or malted red sorghum; extracts like those from white sorghum or brown rice;

caramel malts like buckwheat, millet, or crystal rice; and some small amounts of roasted malts like roasted Goldfinch Millet, roasted Cara Millet, Griffin Millet, or dark Munich millet will help you create all the ideal flavor components in the resulting beer. Boiling the first runnings down to the desired starting gravity is an ideal way to great medal-worthy beer. (Evasion Brewing's Grandpa's Nap barley wine features only Grouse's malted pale millet, with the first runnings from two mashes each collected and boiled down to half of the fermentor's volume).

Mangrove Jack's M15 Empire Ale Yeast or Fermentis SafAle™ S-04 are a common go-to yeasts to employ here. I have noticed certain fruity flavors being elicited by these yeasts; M15 contributing more of a dark fruit character and S-04 a notable earthiness that is common in UK styles. However, you can get similar fruity notes using a slightly different approach and going with Fermentis SafLager™ S-189, which is an alcohol-tolerant lager yeast that produces low amounts of diacetyl, is highly flocculant, does not mind warmer fermentation temperatures, and will help with these fruity notes as well.

Yeast pitching rates are of paramount importance for these stronger styles and, depending on flocculation, you may need to consider a double, triple, or even higher pitch to finish the fermentation completely. High-alcohol styles often run the risk of coming off cloying when not balanced with hops or spices correctly, and that is not helped by the typically higher finishing gravities. Spicy, floral, and fruity hops are advisable, but not so much that they take away from the experience of the rich malt and kettle caramelization, if being included as a feature of the particular style you are brewing. These beers benefit from bottle conditioning, sometimes reaching their peak a year or more after packaging. Unfermentable sugars are crucial to ensure the shelf life and not turn your beer into caramel malt champagne (although that does taste lovely, it will blow up more bottles than it is worth). Aged examples will often present more of a sherry or port-wine-like experience when drinking due to the oxidation that is common with aging.

Commercial examples: Grandpa's Nap, Coastal Colossus (both Evasion Brewing)

PORTER

As there are no dark gluten-free extracts available currently, partial mash or all-grain is the usual approach for gluten-free porters. It takes a deft touch to know how to pepper in darker, roasted malts to draw a clear line, stylistically speaking, for the drinker between brown porter and robust porter. When it comes to the differences between porter and stout, one key difference is the presence of fruity flavors in porter, typically citrus and stone fruit. What can also trip up brewers with porter is the "dryness factor," which in a porter should be largely from finishing gravity and not completely from darker malt astringency.

Brown porter. A gluten-free brown porter recipe would feature base ingredients like sorghum or rice extract, as well as base malts like millet and rice. Although a couple of different lighter colored base grains make complete sense here, there does seem to be some credence to using higher levels of darker malts like those newly available from Grouse's "high dry" program (e.g., dark Munich millet, and darker Vienna millet malts). All these millet and rice options make for good potential base malts specifically because of the clean toasted bread notes and residual sweetness that they contribute. When using high dry malt like Griffin Millet, think toasted raisin bread flavor. This is an important consideration because of the drier finish that brown porter is known for. Using these malts for color and flavor in higher quantities allows for a solid, deep-colored base to layer in a sensible amount of other roasts that will accentuate flavors of deep caramel, licorice, and roast, which can all lean toward to burnt. You could in theory consider any roasts, and it is up to the brewer to blend these with a deft hand to create award-worthy beer. When considering darker rice malts, Eckert's de-hulled versions of dark rice and "Gas Hog" could be a great way to draw the line for the drinker in this style.

Commercial example: Aurochs Porter (Aurochs Brewing Co.)

Robust porter. Although fruity elements are completely to style in any porter, in robust porter there seems to be more attention paid to prominent citrusy flavors, even including specific mention of ingredients like coriander. With that in mind, hops more commonly known for citrus make a lot of sense in a robust porter.

Perceived dryness can come from various factors, but keep in mind that this should be from finishing gravity more so than darker malt astringency, even in robust porter. Thus, while you could theoretically achieve dryness using a yeast like SafAle™ US-05 and a peppering of very dark character malts, you are better off stopping at chocolate roast rather than going even darker. The use of a chocolate malt is also smart because the flavor will likely pair with fruity notes better than flavors like the deeper espresso coffee that can come from darker gluten-free malts.

Commercial examples: 1808 Porter (Burning Brothers Brewing), Baker Street Porter (Bierly Brewing)

COMPARING ROBUST PORTER AND STOUT

The line between porter and stout is often hard to define. Consider brown porter compared with dry Irish stout, which have the same starting and finishing gravity ranges; travel to the Guinness factory and even there they'll say it's hard to tell the difference between a porter and a dry Irish stout. All porters and stouts are opaque, and all of them have roast, chocolate, caramel, or coffee notes permissible by style. The largest difference is the presence of fruity flavors in porters, especially stone fruit and citrus. Robust porter recipes can feature various fruity hops, or even coriander, to achieve noticeable fruit flavors, as well as adjuncts like coffee, cacao nibs, or vanilla. This is due to the lower level of roasted malts in porter compared with stout. Where you might even be able to get away with a little bit of banana flavor in a porter, stouts have almost no fruit esters whatsoever.

The most interesting comparison that can be drawn is when digging into American-style stout categories. One could contend that the American stout style overlaps with robust porter to some degree, as it calls for fruity and citrus aromas and flavors. The largest difference is American stouts call for a distinct dry roast finish, high bitterness and astringency, and a noticeable hop contribution. When designing a robust porter recipe, where sorghum seems to be a common ingredient in gluten-free examples, you can consider achieving fruitiness through syrups with additional roasted grains peppered in. Stout recipes, by contrast, are better when brewed all-grain, as this appears to be the best way to achieve the right "stout-like" qualities. Grains like oats, quinoa, and buckwheat will help lend a fuller mouthfeel when paired with grains like millet and rice in a stout.

STOUT

For most drinkers, roasted barley flavor is what typically denotes a stout, especially in competition categories. From the many gluten-free grains available, you will find it necessary to turn to roast malts like Eckert's dark, "Gas Hog", and Pitch Black rice malts, and Grouse's roasted buckwheat malt, chocolate roast millet, dark roasted millet, and Caramel 240L millet malts. You might get away with using small quantities of these grains in a porter, but specific stout categories should have larger quantities of these very dark roasts, with special attention paid to aspects like darker foam and promoting slightly higher finishing gravities than found in the average porter while still preserving dry roast character. This is especially true when making something like an export stout or sweet stout, as the roast will help balance the residual sweetness that is characteristic of these styles. No matter what, a layering of additional medium roasts and unmalted grains and adjuncts to provide additional body and smoothness will help you stay true to style when crafting a gluten-free stout.

Dry Irish stout. Thanks to the brewing juggernaut that is Guinness, dry Irish stout is likely most beer drinkers' first impression of a stout. There is often a smoothness that is described as a creamy character in some guidelines but not others, and may not actually be as appropriate as it would be in other stout categories. Coffee flavors and a dry finish are important, as the flavors should not linger on the pallet. These beers are noticeably lower in alcohol than other stout styles; while some commercial versions may be a little higher in ABV, their dry finish puts them into this category. Since this is a dryer style, you will likely want to focus on enzymatic contact times and stay away from caramel malts and similar ingredients.

Commercial examples: Moka Diosa Stout (Divine Science Brewing), TantaMount Stout (Evasion Brewing), No Doubt Stout (Two Bays Brewing Co.), Glutenberg Stout (Glutenberg)

Export stout. Export stouts are typified by coffee, roasted malt aroma, some acidity and astringency but with body and sweetness, a higher ABV than dry stout, and persistent head retention. Higher ABV aside, this category has specific notes about more body and sweetness that distinguishes it from dry Irish stout, although the two styles are strikingly similar in description and guidelines. Just bear in mind that neither dry Irish stout nor export stout should be confused with a sweet stout or specialty stout.

With export stout, you can follow many of the suggestions from dry Irish stout when selecting base and roast malts, but this style may also benefit from some deeper caramel malts (like the caramel millet malts from Grouse) to lend a bit of sweetness. You will likely want to have your enzymes in contact with the mash for less time to elicit a higher finishing gravity—this will also mean that you will need to use more malt than with a dry Irish stout.

Commercial examples: Watchstander Stout (Ghostfish Brewing Company), Riva Stout (Holidaily Brewing Co.), Blackbird Stout (Bierly Brewing)

Imperial stout. Imperial stouts are rich and malty, with high finishing gravities usually between 1.020 and 1.030. For a gluten-free imperial stout, this will mean either using back-sweetening as a strategy or carefully selecting malt and adjuncts to achieve a high finishing gravity. Base malts like Grouse's millet and buckwheat malts naturally make good choices, and the various rice malts from Eckert will help with both sugar extraction and color.

American versions of imperial stout tend to have higher levels of fruity esters. Therefore, I suggest adding sorghum syrup to the recipe to boost starting gravity and lend a noticeable fruit note in an American version of a gluten-free imperial stout, but I do not recommend this for a British version of the same. When brewing a British version and your brewing system limits mash tun space, I recommend double or triple batching into your fermentor to achieve the correct volume with an appropriately high starting gravity.

You can also consider exposing the mash to your enzymes for a shorter time to ensure a higher finishing gravity. Adding ample amounts of maltodextrin is another way to boost the final gravity and increase fullness in the mouth.

Commercial examples: Santa's Nightcap (Holidaily Brewing Co.), Imperial Darkness and Kantankerous Stout (Ground Breaker Brewing), Batch 2 Barrel Aged Imperial Stout (Evasion Brewing), Hella Nibs (Otherwise Brewing)

BELGIAN AND FRENCH ALE

Bière de garde. For bière de garde, the color needs to be light amber to chestnut brown/red and the taste characterized by slight toasted malt notes and sweetness. This is a great beer style in which to use Grouse's roasted millet malts, such as Dutch Roast, Red Wing, roasted Cara Millet, and roasted Goldfinch. You can go clean or use a wild yeast like *Brettanomyces* with this style, but high levels of Brett character will pull this out of style. Although bière de garde has its root in French farmhouse brewing, this style typically has a cleaner finish since it was brewed during the colder months. As such, sorghum (syrup and malted), malted and unmalted millet, rice malt, buckwheat (malted and unmalted), and flaked quinoa could all be ingredients when approaching this style gluten free. Bière de garde is a style that has a fair amount of leeway when it comes to ABV (4%–8%) but it should not be all the way dried out. What makes this style special is the balance of the residual body and sweetness melded with the toasted malt notes, which makes for an incredible experience. Even without farmhouse flavors being dominant, you can still bring fruity flavors and acidity to the table through various techniques because of the latitude this style allows for.

Commercial examples: Bière Du Divin (Divine Science Brewing), Yamhill Punch 2021 (Evasion Brewing)

Classic saison. The classic saison has a yeast-driven flavor profile and is expected to be on the dry side and have low body. Esters and phenols are common flavors, with spicy black pepper and fruit dominating the overall impression. Saison is a lovely style with which you can use just about any gluten-free grain bill. If thinking about competing with a gluten-free saison, you may want to consider that a specialty saison category might be a better place to have your unique grains stand out. Since a specialty category usually requires you to write in your ingredients, all those specialty ingredients will not be seen as off-flavors when tasted in a line-up (if properly used, of course).

Speaking of pepper flavors, flaked quinoa and malted buckwheat have been present in my favorite gluten-free versions of this style, as they seem to contain the perfect precursors for a saison yeast strain to elicit amazing complementary flavors of pink peppercorn as well as white and black pepper. Despite saison yeast drying the beer out, the high protein levels in quinoa and buckwheat can help increase body and head retention, which heightens the experience and will get you closer to the mark. For some great added flavor and character, Red Wing millet malt from Grouse or amber rice malt from Eckert make sense in limited amounts.

Commercial example: 7 Grain Saison (Moonshrimp Brewing)

Belgian-style oud bruin. Although it is rare to find oud bruin in gluten-free form, when you find it, get it. If you cannot get it, definitely brew it yourself. A darker colored sour that ranges from slightly to highly acidic (it can even be acetic at times) and can offer roast notes from low to high, oud bruin offers some stylistic leeway and is a great option for the gluten-free brewer who wants to make a sour. To build a recipe like this, I would favor base grains like millet, rice, and sorghum, and factor in using character malts like roasted millet, rice and buckwheat to achieve this style. Grouse's medium roast, Dutch Roast, roasted Cara Millet, dark Munich millet, and Griffin Millet are all great character malts in an oud bruin.

Using a lactic acid-producing yeast is a smart choice, with the flavors developing as the beer matures. To be true to the style, it is not recommended to kettle sour with bacteria, but this technique could in theory be employed. Additionally, a clean wood character blended with all of these other flavors makes for a world-class experience, although it is not necessary. If you are planning to use wood, make sure it is neutral, as spirit or wine-influenced tastes from the wood are not to style.

Commercial examples: Dark Sour (Beliveau Farms)

Belgian-style dubbel. A Belgian-style dubbel can be achieved with base malts and syrups like millet, rice, and sorghum, but it is the character malts that truly make this style. Belgian dubbels are brown to very dark, with cocoa, dark and dried fruit flavors, and a noticeable yeast phenolic spice character. For some character and color, darker caramel and Red Wing millet malts from Grouse or James' Brown Rice and crystal rice malts from Eckert make sense in a dubbel. Banana, cherry, and other fruit flavors coming from the yeast are more subdued in this style but will be present. The biggest thing to focus on in a dubbel is head retention and tight bubble formation, as style guidelines suggest mousse-like foam; bottle conditioning or higher carbonation (in addition to high-protein malts) helps with this, as do adjuncts like lentils. Candi syrup is typically a go-to for most brewers, but not completely necessary. In fact, too much candi syrup can compete with the character malts. That said, syrups are a great choice, the main reason to use them being to make sure you hit the right ABV and color, and to stress the yeast to help enhance desirable aromas and flavors.

Commercial examples: Dubbel (Bierly Brewing), Endeavor (Green's), Abbey Dubbel (Mutantis)

Belgian-style tripel. Belgian-style tripels are definitely where light syrups make sense, specifically because of how well-attenuated this beer style is known to be, though you may choose to balance against this to maximize protein content and head retention in the overall beer. Malted oats make some sense in this beer style, but only as a character malt—for base malts you will need to look to grains like rice and sorghum that have much higher extract potentials in order to hit the high ABV expected of this style. The complexity and fruitiness can in theory be approached from a couple of angles, so decide if you want that contribution to come from a more complex grain bill, primarily from the yeast, or from a more even mix of malt and yeast character. At any rate, most available dry yeasts have alcohol tolerances that fall into tripel territory. You can brew a tripel with all rice, all sorghum, or all millet, but the best characteristics will be achieved when you pepper in some additional buckwheat or quinoa.

Commercial examples: Quest (Green's), Go Big or Go Home (Departed Soles Brewing Co.)

GERMAN-STYLE KÖLSCH

Whereas a blonde ale style can feature many grains, a to-style gluten-free Kölsch should be based on millet, rice, and, in some cases, sorghum, to achieve the specific tastes that are acceptable for this category. There should be no vegetal notes nor fruity notes in this style, which is why malt is much more advisable than syrup if using sorghum as a base ingredient. There are times when pear wine–like tastes can be acceptable in this style, but only if mildly perceptible. Some oat malt can be used to achieve lasting foam, which is to style, but not so much that a caramel taste is communicated (around 2% of the grain bill and you should be fine). To add great foam without compromising on clean taste, Grouse's caramel buckwheat or raw millet could be considered. Grouse's Cara Millet and Goldfinch millet malts are great ways to add a bready note. You can add a little bit of gypsum for extra crispness in this style, as well as some calcium chloride for more malt expression and to balance hop perception. This style also benefits from a lower pH, and many barley-based examples include some acidulated malt; unfortunately, acidulated malt is not currently available to gluten-free brewers unless you make it yourself.

Commercial examples: Kolsch (Buck Wild Brewing), Sprutz Kölsch (Evasion Brewing)

AMERICAN LIGHT LAGER

American lager is a style that literally has gluten-free grains built into it! Why not use them the whole way through? Sorghum will dry out well, but might lend too many fruity esters to be in style. Rice, corn, millet, sweet potato, even demerara sugar can conceivably be used as recipe components. In fact, an American lager recipe with an equal blending of all five of these ingredients would make a commendable beer—a good boil and well-executed diacetyl rest will leave you with an incredibly crisp and refreshing lager. When force carbonating in a keg, be aggressive and shoot for 2.7–2.9 volumes of CO_2.

Making an American light lager is a great idea once you have mastered some other lager styles like Pilsner and helles. Gluten-free grains help a brewer achieve a low-calorie and low-carb beer; using the right enzymes will help your beer consistently finish below 1.000 standard gravity. Rice, sweet potato, corn, and millet are all great selections here for providing clean fermentables. Mashing above 175°F (79.4°C) for at least an hour with the necessary exogenous enzymes is advisable to create a high-glucose wort.

Commercial examples: Light Lager (Evasion Brewing), Aurochs Light Lager (Aurochs Brewing Co.)

PILSNER

Pilsner is a beer style rich in history, intrigue, and global sales. As I discussed in chapter 2, to call a gluten-free lager a "Pilsner" is actually rather incongruous considering no Pilsner barley malt is used. Gluten-free styles like this place a tremendous weight on wort and yeast stewardship—even more so than in the barley-based versions—with clean, crisp taste and subtle noble hop flavors and aromas singing perfectly together in harmony. Achieving a gluten-free "Pilsner" takes different techniques and careful consideration of ingredients.

American-style Pilsner. Certain guidelines state that the grain bill for an American Pilsner must be 25% corn or rice, but you could conceivably use 50% corn and 50% rice for the grain bill and make a wonderful interpretation of a gluten-free American Pilsner. While this would undoubtedly make a refreshingly crisp beer, you do run the risk of fermenting all the way to 1.000 specific gravity, so adding maltodextrin or raw grains is advised if using primarily rice and corn. Outside of corn and rice, whichever gluten-free base malt you have available will likely do the trick. American Pilsners are differentiated from traditional Pilsners by heavier hopping, with a noticeable American hop note (Cluster, Willamette, Brewer's Gold, etc.).

Commercial examples: New Grist (Lakefront Brewery), Redbridge (Anheuser-Busch), Enterprise Dry Hopped Lager (Green's)

International-style Pilsner. As with American-style Pilsners, international-style Pilsners should use high amounts of adjunct. With very little bitterness at all, balance is everything in these beers; they should lean malty and be crystal clear. Typical base malts are millet and rice but there is some more leeway if considering Pilsners not from Asia. Although Japanese-inspired rice lager makes a ton of sense for this category, and all-rice beers can taste amazing, you could in theory make an African-inspired sorghum lager and still be in style in this category. Elements like lasting foam are still important here—since sorghum and rice are not known for lasting head retention unless special considerations are made, both grains typically need to be used in malted form and with special enzymatic treatments. You might also think about ingredients that help as foam stabilizers, like unmalted millet or buckwheat.

Commercial examples: Calrose Crisp (Otherwise Brewing), Circuit Breaker Lager (Suspect Brewing)

German-style Pilsner. German-style Pilsners are malty and sweet, with light bread and biscuit notes, but also dry and crisp. A German-style Pilsner will have a lower finishing gravity than a Munich-style helles, the latter having more residual sugars and dextrins. Millet and rice are good choices for gluten-free German-style Pilsner. Nailing the persistent head is important, so using maltodextrin may be advisable if your base malt won't do the job. It may benefit from the use of oat malt but in very small quantities so as to not elicit too much caramel or haze. Late hopping is fine, but do not use dry hopping.

Commercial examples: 10-09 German Pilsner (Rolling Mill Brewing Co.), Felix Pilsener (Bierly Brewing), Lager (Two Bays Brewing Co.)

Bohemian-style Pilsner. Having a higher finishing gravity than even Munich-style helles, Bohemian-style Pilsner also features much stronger toasted bread, caramel, and biscuit flavors and a more pronounced noble hop character. Saaz hops are to style here. Low levels of diacetyl and sulfur can be present, but not offensively so. Pale millet malt, biscuit rice, and pale rice are all great choices for base malts, with some additional depth of flavor achieved through character malts like Munich or Vienna. A thick, rocky head is advisable, so raw millet, caramel buckwheat, and pale oat malt can help you achieve all of these characteristics in a gluten-free version; there is also the option of adding maltodextrin.

Commercial examples: Divine Millsner (Divine Science Brewing)

AMBER LAGER

German-style Märzen. Märzen is a mid-strength lager with straw to deep gold coloring. Grouse's pale millet malt and Eckert's 4°L biscuit rice malt are likely your two best choices for base malts. Munich millet malt also recommends itself as a base malt for this style—Munich millet is a better choice here than Vienna millet due to the caramel and toffee notes Vienna can elicit. No caramel should be present in this style. Using a malt like Eckert's crystal rice will give you clean sweetness, but caramel millet malts should be avoided because they contribute a much more noticeable caramel note. Some light roast millet, roasted Cara Millet, and Goldfinch Millet are great character malts here. To be to-style, noble hops should be used in a German Märzen.

Commercial examples: James Märzen (Bierly Brewing), Märzen Attacks (Ghostfish Brewing Company)

American-style Oktoberfest. Caramel and roast malts are on the table for the American-style Oktoberfest. The caramel should be secondary to a bready and biscuity taste, so consider Eckert's 5°L biscuit rice malt, alongside Grouse's Munich millet and caramel millet malts. A small peppering of Cara Millet could be used to get a toasted bread taste. While this style is still a lager, there could be a noticeable noble hop character that is more pronounced than its German cousin.

Commercial examples: Amber Lager (Ground Breaker Brewing), Oktoberfest (Holidaily)

Vienna lager. Vienna lagers are copper to reddish brown and characterized by a malty aroma and sweetness on the palate with a light toast note to balance. Higher-sulfate waters may contribute a nice crisp note, as will a peppering of grains like malted rice to your recipe. Grouse's Vienna millet malt comes directly to mind as a base malt for a gluten-free version of this style. The Vienna millet may lend too much toffee flavor by itself, however, so you will need to cut that flavor with pale millet malt and unmalted millet, as well as add character malts like a darker Munich millet, light roast millet, and Goldfinch Millet (also available from Grouse). The flavor should be clean, with no fruit notes, so certain grains like sorghum will not make sense for this style, and neither will grains that contribute spicy tastes and aromas like pale buckwheat and flaked quinoa.

Commercial examples: Vienna Lager (Holidaily Brewing Co.), Ganz Vienna Lager (Bierly Brewing)

BOCK

Bock. Brewing all-malt is important in a bock, although you can achieve a higher ABV by using either sorghum or brown rice syrup. Base malts like pale millet, Vienna and Munich millet malts, and biscuit rice and pale rice malts all make sense here. Malt, sweet, nutty, and some toast flavors can be present in a bock, but no caramel should be noticeable.

The GABF 2021 style guidelines say the color should range from dark brown to very dark. This is a special consideration when brewing gluten-free beer, since many of the darker roast and caramel gluten-free malts give a toffee or caramel note even in small quantities, which would easily push your beer out of style. This means that you will need to balance these flavors by focusing on malts that have been kilned for longer rather than roasted to achieve their color. Light roast and chocolate roast millet malts are potential ingredients as the light roast can lend nuttiness, but the chocolate may lend too much astringency. Grouse's dark Munich millet and Griffin Millet malts may be better choices to elicit the desired flavors, with dark Munich contributing toasted bread and bran notes, and Griffin Millet toffee and pumpernickle aromas and flavors. You really only need to use bittering hops (e.g., Magnum) in a beer like this since hop aroma is not to style.

Commercial examples: While there is not a commercial example of a gluten-free bock (or, indeed, a Maibock), it is a cherished style for me.

Maibock. Maibock is a pale to light amber style of bock, with at most a slight toasted bread taste. Biscuit rice and pale and Munich millet make sense for base malts, as do syrups (syrups help reach the higher starting gravities). Maibock leans slightly drier than the bock category, but you will still look to finishing gravities above 1.012. This is another style in which Grouse's Goldfinch Millet Malt works well as a character malt, as would a small amount of Red Wing Millet (also Grouse) or amber rice malt (Eckert). There should be noble hop character in the aroma but very little perceived bitterness in the taste, so you will need to use much less hops, or a smaller, more continuous hopping method, to truly make this style sing.

Doppelbock. Doppelbock is a rich, high-alcohol lager with incredible flavors and aromas permissible. It is also a touch darker and will likely come out copper to dark brown. This is a style where toffee, caramel, plum, and raisin are completely to style, so peppering in character malts like Grouse's caramel millet malts, Griffin Millet, and roasted Cara Millet alongside Eckert's crystal, James' Brown, and darker biscuit rice malts makes a ton of sense here. I wouldn't say that there is a right or wrong base malt in this style, but the focus should be on maximizing your starting gravity, with the intention that the beer should not ferment all the way. In fact, it is common in this style for gravities to finish between 1.014 and 1.020. I have seen National Homebrewer's competition results where a winning doppelbock finished with a gravity of 1.045! I thought to myself, "I could literally make a whole additional beer with that gravity . . ."

Commercial examples: Ghostfish 5th Anniversary Doppelbock (Ghostfish Brewing Company)

DARK LAGER

Czech dark lager. From copper to black, the Czech style of dark lager calls for anywhere from a little roast to a lot, but this style is best known for a deep maltiness and higher hop perception, with finishing gravities around 1.014–1.018. Some diacetyl and stone fruit character is admissible, but only pleasantly so. Good options for gluten-free base malts include Eckert's biscuit and pale rice malts, or Grouse's pale or Munich millet malts. Chocolate millet malt and even a small dosing of dark rice or dark millet malt make sense as character malts, but you can likely achieve a more to-style beer by employing Grouse's Dutch Roast and medium roast millet malts as well as the deeper biscuit rice malts available from Eckert, the latter especially useful if you are aiming on the lower side of roasted notes. Roasted buckwheat, when used in the right quantity, as well as some raw millet can aid in foam retention and help boost residual sugars. A gluten-free brewer approaching this style might also try to put more complex sugars into the wort using techniques discussed in chapter 5, as well as having maltodextrin on hand to ensure a higher finishing gravity if needed.

Commercial examples: Gluten-free versions of Czech-style dark lagers tend to be limited releases, and I do not know of one currently on the shelves at time of writing; however, there is a Czech dark lager recipe in chapter 7.

American dark lager. In contrast to Czech-style dark lager, caramel is more appropriate in the American dark lager style. Another distinction in American dark lager is the low body and high carbonation. Munich Millet and biscuit rice malts make sense as base malts, and Griffin Millet and Vienna millet (including the various roast versions Grouse can offer) all make tremendous amounts of sense as character malts for achieving this style. Grains like the dark caramel millet malts (e.g., Caramel 90L, 120L, and 240L from Grouse), roasted buckwheat, dark roasted rice (150°L), dark roasted millet malt, chocolate millet malt, and even dark candi syrups are all good choices to provide roast caramel flavors in an American dark lager, but use them sparingly to achieve the darker and more caramel tastes, otherwise they will come to dominate the beer.

Commercial examples: Tall Dark and Roasted (Holidaily Brewing Company).

TRADITIONAL OR HISTORICAL STYLES

I am including a broad description of some important traditional and historical styles in this chapter for completeness. By their nature, these beers are gluten free and, thus, we are not concerned with using gluten-free ingredients to emulate a barley or wheat-based drink. Of course, the grains to use will be self-evident, so this discussion will focus more on other stylistic aspects.

In competition guidelines, the traditional and historical categories typically mention beers like chicha and African sorghum beer—basically any traditional style that cannot be placed with a modern or historical barley-based category. The broad sweep of beers covered by such categories illustrates how few options non-barley-based beers have outside a designated "gluten-free" category when entered into competitions. While using historically relevant brewing techniques can have a tremendous amount of merit for brewers either looking for a tasty, refreshing beverage or seeking a podium finish, it is possible to produce accomplished renditions of "traditional and historical" (i.e., non-barley) beers with modern mashing techniques like the use of exogenous enzymes. Brews like African sorghum or millet beer (of which there are several, but I'll refer to them with the catchall "African beer" for the sake of brevity) and Peruvian chicha are essentially brewed to be sour; as such, there are a couple of different ways to approach this, both traditionally and with a modern take.

A common method that is key to achieving the tart to sour note characteristic of African beers is a version of a kettle sour that is done pre-boil. This involves a long overnight mash after the crushed grains are added to warm water; this employs the natural microflora present on the grains to lower the wort pH, aid in wort fermentability, and elicit flavors and aromas that come through in the finished beer. The following day, the steeped grains are heated, then the liquid is separated from the grain and boiled.

For a style like chicha, sourcing *Pichia* yeast species for a secondary or co-fermentation is necessary to nail the unique flavor of this style. That is not to say that you couldn't come close using lactic acid producing co-fermentations that feature yeast and bacteria. I've tried chicha recipes that were fermented with saison yeast and didn't end up tart—while that makes for a lovely interpretation of the style, the lack of traditional chicha flavor means it won't have all the makings of a medal-winning beer in the traditional and historical category.

Additional modern brewing techniques like using hops, while seemingly complementary to the robust flavors of many traditional beers, are not to style and could be counterproductive at the judging table when competing in a historical category. A careful explanation should be given when entering a beer with these elements. (This is not just for non-European styles either—for example, a historical style that specifically neglects hops is gruit.) You can use just about anything else that is historically relevant to add bitterness and astringency in such styles, but not hops—hop aromas and tastes featured in this style will most certainly keep you from the podium.

Commercial examples: Chicha Morada and Pulque Metztli (Dos Luces Brewery), Gruit (Moonshrimp Brewing)

Take every chance to play with styles and various brewing techniques. We only covered a small percentage of the known styles out there, and there are still so many to explore. Go forth and brew a style, no matter what—just know that, when it comes to competitions and recognition is on the line, specific malts are better and more to style than others because of their specific flavor contributions.

Even still, there are many styles left to be created, and I anticipate many of those will include gluten-free grains like millet, buckwheat, quinoa, and sorghum as well as grains that already exist in barley categories, like oats, rice, and corn. The reason being is that their unique contributions to beer flavor demand categories other than "specialty" or "experimental" as their flavors are more fully understood at this point.

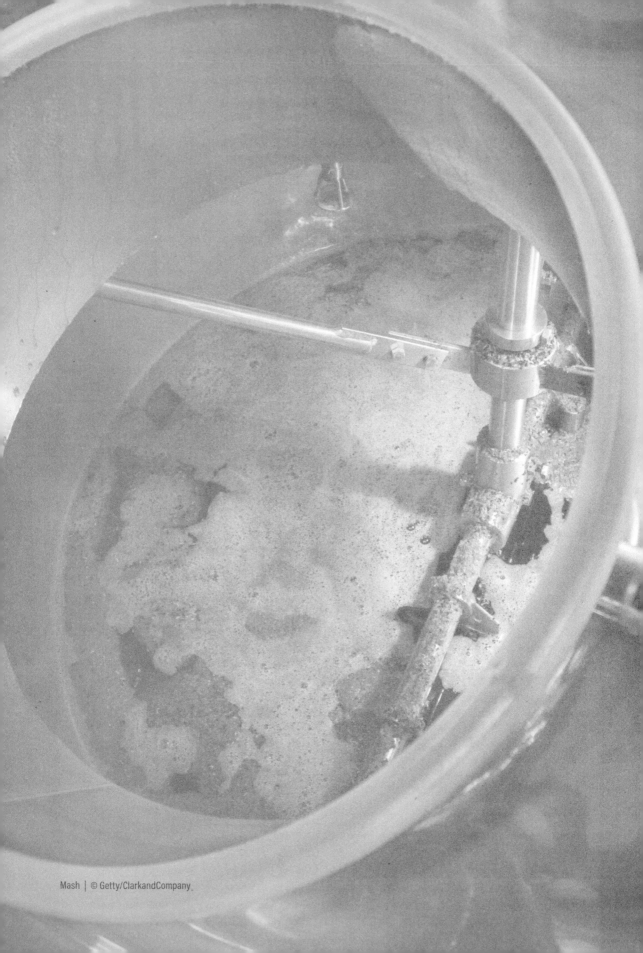

5

Mashing Techniques

In this chapter, we will briefly look at some of the high-level concepts behind mashing, which will set the context to then discuss the philosophy of gluten-free mashing and mention some relevant research done on the subject. Brewers may have their options dictated by the brew systems they have invested in, so we'll look at various mash methods that can be employed depending on the existing setup. There is also a "getting started" section for homebrewers who are looking into the ideal home brewhouse setup suitable for their gluten-free endeavors. Then we will look at the enzymes available to use for homebrewers and professional brewers, which will include endogenous enzymes (i.e., those enzymes naturally occurring in the grain) as well as commercially available exogenous enzyme products that are invaluable aids in gluten-free brewing. We will then break down various mash regimes, focusing on the specific rest temperatures and times that ensure proper enzymatic activity during a given stage of the mash.

In the context of modern brewing methods, gluten-free brewing is an area still in its infancy. There is no consensus among gluten-free brewers as to the "go-to" mash regime, so there is no "one true method" you can apply to a specific beer style that can be brewed gluten free. We should also acknowledge the fact that people have been making gluten-free beers for a long, long time. As we saw in chapter 1, before barley became the de facto brewing grain across the world thanks to colonialism and, latterly, globalization, brewers in all parts of the world were making gluten-free beer that was just . . . beer. Those brewers used whatever worked and whatever was easiest to source in their part of the world. I encourage you to keep this in mind when you are reading about the many, seemingly unfamiliar, ingredients and techniques discussed in this book: do what works for you, based on the system and grains you have. With the many different grains you can choose and types of mash regime you can employ, plus a few other tweaks here and there, you can achieve a whole host of different and delicious flavors, including making a beer that is almost completely identical to its barley cousin.

OVERVIEW OF MASHING

A beer brewer uses malted grains, typically barley, because of the enzymes that are intrinsic to grain that is malted. These enzymes are synthesized within the grain during the germination process; if left to continue, under suitable conditions, that grain grows into a plant. The maltster starts this germination process, but ends it after a short time with kilning; provided the kilning treatment is not too hot, as is the case with base malts, the malted grains retain these newly synthesized enzymes, making them available to the brewer when mashing to create various sweet worts that yeast can ferment into beer.

The two enzymes with which brewers are probably most familiar are α-amylase (alpha-amylase) and β-amylase (beta-amylase). Both are present in malted barley in relatively high amounts, but gluten-free malts contain much lower levels and some lack one or the other amylase altogether (Ledley et al. 2021, 9). Starch consists of very (very!) long chains made from individual glucose molecules joined together; these chains are also branched to varying degrees, allowing the starch molecules to grow to great lengths within the confines of the barley kernel. The enzymatic activity of the two amylases breaks the bonds that hold together most of the individual sugar units in starch, releasing a mix of simpler sugars into the wort. These sugars consist largely of glucose, maltose (which consists of two glucose molecules joined together), maltotriose (three glucose molecules), and maltotetraose (you guessed it, four glucose molecules). Yeast eats sugars like these during fermentation, especially maltose and glucose, generating mostly alcohol and carbon dioxide as a result. These sugars and the amylases that create them are necessary for making beer, but many other enzymes are involved in the biochemical reactions of the mash and help improve the quality of the resulting beverage.

Barley also contains enzymes called limit dextrinase and α-glucosidase, which break apart specific bonds where the starch chains form branch points. Amylases cannot break apart sugars close to these branch points, so there is a limit to how much of the total starch α- and β-amylase can convert into simple sugars. The result is lots of carbohydrate molecules of variable length containing branch points, known as limit dextrins. The activity of limit dextrinase and, to a lesser extent, α-glucosidase is important because it works to break the branch points in both starch and limit dextrins. Once these branch points have been removed, the amylases can work at creating more fermentable sugars. The number of limit dextrins left in the wort is dependent upon the quantity and activity of the limit dextrinase, and this in turn is dependent upon the conditions of the mash. As most brewer's yeast strains cannot ferment limit dextrins, any that remain in the wort after fermentation can lend additional sweetness, body, and mouthfeel to the resulting beer, which is highly desirable in many beer styles. Many gluten-free malts actually possess higher levels of limit dextrinase than barley malt.

Barley also contains enzymes like proteases, which break down proteins and peptides, and lipases, which break down fats (lipids). And don't forget about pentosanases, cellulases, and β-glucanase! Between them, the various activities of these enzymes aid in foam stability and head retention, affect wort viscosity, and help create aqueous free amino nitrogen that is essential for yeast health, among other things.

For the mash itself, the brewer crushes the malted grain to make the starches accessible and adds them to warm or hot water to liquify these starches and cause gelatinization, which is a physical process that happens in grains at various temperatures where the starches are degraded or unraveled and can then be worked on by the various enzymes. As we will discuss below, while there are some similarities to mashing with barley, many gluten-free grains have special considerations because of the various chemical differences between them and barley. As mentioned in chapter 2, these differences include issues such as little to no endogenous enzymatic activity, different gelatinization temperatures, and smaller grain size.

Do not be daunted by these differences, for research has shown that certain gluten-free grains do contain many of these enzymes, and even if a brewer does not have access to exogenous enzymes, brewing strategies can still be used that will create excellent beer. For the brewer who *does* have access to exogenous enzymes, you will have to consider which enzymes you need to add based on the system you're using, its capabilities, and how it will handle your choice of grains.

BREWHOUSE CONSIDERATIONS

EQUIPMENT

There are a lot of factors that contribute to a successful brew day: as well as recipe formulation, there is the equipment you use.

In a commercial context, equipment considerations will be based on the existing system. Bear in mind that most brewhouses at any scale are made with specifications for barley. This may present certain challenges but it is generally possible to make things work, it all depends on what you have at your disposal. For example, many pro brewers recommend a separate cereal cooker if you plan on using certain grains that require higher temperature mashes, which applies to many gluten-free grains, but many brewhouses have a hot liquor tank set up so that the brewing liquor can be heated up to boiling if need be.

Holidaily Brewing Company, a dedicated gluten-free brewery, has taken a further step to increase efficiencies by using mash press filter system. These systems begin with a finer and more consistent grist, achieved using a hammer mill, and a constantly stirred mash slurry for greater enzymatic efficiency. This mash slurry is then pumped into an accordion-like mash press filter, where the slurry is divided into 40+ individual chambers. In these chambers, the mash is compressed against a fine filter screen using air bladders, sparged with fresh water, and compressed again to extract as much usable sugar from the grain as possible.

Since most breweries do not have such a system at their disposal, the mash screen can be a stumbling block when starting out with gluten-free brewing. Even with a false bottom modification you will likely still have grain pieces that squeeze through into the boil kettle, or they can be just small enough to get caught in the screen and not allow any liquid to pass. As with all-grain brewing in general, the secret is setting up the mash bed properly. Stirring the mash at the beginning and for the enzymatic additions (rakes or a stirring element can be used at scale), then stopping the stirring and continuing with vorlauf seem to be a best for ensuring proper incorporation of the enzymes and drainage. When there are still concerns over drainage, you can always fall back on rice hulls, but in many brewhouses this is an "overspend" and not truly necessary, as consistent sugar extraction without wort channeling appears to be a problem that can be solved enzymatically. If certain compounds like β-glucan are not processed by the enzymes then you may still encounter a stuck mash, which is why rice hulls can still be a good fail-safe and help with brew day peace of mind. Grains like millet are all so small and similar in size that they can get stuck themselves, even without containing compounds like β-glucan. This is where knowledge of the contents of your brewing grains and malts makes a huge difference on brew day.

At the homebrewing level, I regularly find myself reaching for one piece of kitchen equipment: a fine mesh strainer with a handle. The reason for the mesh strainer is that I can pick up any excess grain particles that make their way into the boil kettle. Even then, many grain elements like the husk may make it into the boil kettle. Many may be concerned with extracting tannins, but from my experience this has seemingly never negatively impacted the resulting flavor of the downstream beer. This issue can be exacerbated by improper pH. A safe target for mash strike water before mash-in is pH 5.2–5.6 depending on the enzymes you are using. You can of course dial it in from there, but pH in this range will help prevent you from extracting too many unpleasant tannic compounds into the finished beer. It also corresponds with the range in which many enzymes, exogenous and endogenous, appear to work best.

Another pro-tip that I recommend for homebrewers is to do some of the water treatments (salts and acid) before adding the malt, which may help you when looking to mash in on the hotter side. Doing this will make sure you do not extract tannic off-flavors during brewing, as many gluten-free methods recommend an initial strike water temperature above 170°F (76.7°C), which is certainly not common practice in brewing with barley.

HOMEBREW EQUIPMENT: GETTING STARTED

Whether you're a stovetop, all-in-one, or mash cooler homebrewer, there will be things in gluten-free brewing that you can pull off a fair bit easier with the right equipment. Gluten-free brewers are generally happy to help share their findings and give advice, so you should also look to ask questions of the community if you need help (e.g., https://www.facebook.com/groups/ZeroToleranceGF/).

A quick caveat for the prospective gluten-free brewer. As referenced previously, many systems are designed for barley-specific brewing conditions. While certain retailers may sell things like wire mesh or other filter screens, you may need to modify your false bottom regardless of the mash tun you choose. Millet, quinoa, and other small grain pieces sneaking into your boil kettle can be annoying, but all of those grains slipping through your screen would make for a tough brew day as you would have to have a recovery strategy on how to separate your grains from the brewing liquid. Setting up your grain bed is an important step and can present some difficulties with too porous of a false bottom.

Stove Top Brewing

Using a stove top is probably the fastest way for beginners to start brewing beer, but there are some restrictions to consider. For example, you will only be able to fit about a 3–4-gallon (11.4–15.1 L) stock pot comfortably on most conventional stoves, which nets your about 32 to 36 twelve-ounce bottles of beer. Maybe that feels like more than enough, but trust me, somehow you'll always be running out of beer. The strength of your burner—gas, coil, or electric—could also lead to some scorching. Although brew-in-a-bag (BIAB) is a common way to do partial or all-grain brewing, it is still an imperfect way to separate the grain from the liquid. Controlling temperature for the duration of the mash will likely be difficult, so plan to have something to insulate the pot, or, if the pot fits, you could leave it sitting covered in a warm oven (preheated to 175°F, or 80°C, and turned off). At any rate, a remote thermometer or something that can handle extreme heat like an oven thermometer will help in making sure you hit and hold your rest temperatures. You could even consider a crock pot as a potential mashing resource, but you will need an adjustable temperature control to achieve the best mashes with that sort of device, and you will of course be limited on size. A truly great tool to consider for stove top brewing is a sous vide machine, as knowing the true temperature of the water and step-mashing up or down in temperature is basically taken care of for you. For this method, you will want to at least wrap some sort of fine mesh around the sous vide tray for easier cleaning, and have a strategy for separating the grains from the sugary wort, for which you could use a brewing bag.

If going stove top is the quickest way for you to get started with brewing, then get started! Additionally, most beginner recipes are all-extract, so you really don't have to worry too much about the all-grain or partial mash considerations just yet.

You will want to also figure out a bigger bowl or bucket to cool your boil kettle in. This will also help hot break materials and other elements settle out to the bottom and ensure a great tasting beer downstream. You might feel like you are too small scale for this, but get an auto siphon too—it makes getting the wort into your fermentor much faster, and will typically leave your floor a lot less sticky.

Mash Cooler with Separate Boil Kettle

This setup is based on the classic commercial setup of a single infusion mash tun, though in this case milled grains are added to brewing water (brewing liquor) that is heated to strike temperature and stirred to achieve mash temperature—in a commercial setup, the grains and water are added simultaneously. For gluten-free brewing, this setup can come with trade-offs. Methods like rising temperature step mashes are quite difficult—depending on the ones you use, many enzymes (e.g., Ondea® Pro) will denature if the water you use to raise the temperature is too hot. A mash cooler is, however, perfectly suited to do a falling temperature step mash, and if all-grain brewing is your route, this will get you going quickly. Kits for converting off-the-shelf Igloo® coolers are relatively inexpensive and you can be small-batch brewing quickly. The relatively low cost of these mash vessels can make brewing gluten-free in a separate, dedicated vessel not such a difficult decision to make if, say, you also brew with barley.

Many of the same best practices in barley brewing can apply in gluten-free brewing, such as recirculating your mash liquid, otherwise known as vorlauf. Homebrewers can of course add a pump to this set up to increase throughput and brewhouse efficiency by shortening mash times.

You will not be able to boil in the mash cooler. This can be incorporated into a stove top setup or a gas or electric boil element.

All-in-One Homebrew System

An all-in-one system, such as the Grainfather, is often a worthy investment for gluten-free brewing if you have the budget, because there really aren't too many limitations. One thing to note is that you will be lucky if you can brew more than one beer in a day on an all-in-one system, but they are available in larger sizes, typically between 5 and 60 US gallons (19–227 L), so you get more yield from your time and effort. Whether falling or rising temperatures or a single-temperature infusion, these systems can handle it, and on top of that fit conveniently into small areas since there is not a separate vessel required to do things like heat brewing water or boil, whirlpool, and chill wort. A pulley mechanism lifts the mash vessel up and above the kettle below, which is also the boil kettle. Hot sparge and lauter water is added and gravity does the rest until the proper volume is collected into the boil kettle. You will need a smaller vessel to heat sparge/lauter liquid, but the usual American five-gallon homebrew batch only involves 2–3 gal. of sparge liquor (about 7.5–11.4 L for a 19 L batch), depending on the strike volume and water absorption rates of various grains. The big downside of some of these systems is that they are electric and so often take longer to achieve a boil—at least, they do if you live in North America or another region with 110-volt mains electricity. Be cognizant of this when buying an all-in-one system; while the household dryer outlet in many American homes will let you run a device using 220 volts, many apartments and smaller houses might not have this capability. However, various larger versions of these systems are made that use natural gas, often marketed as pilot or nano systems.

Multi-vessel Brewing

This is the system that is basically a miniature version of a professional setup. It is also recommended for ideal throughput. Although you'll have to dedicate more space for brewing, you can brew up to four beers or more in a day when you add more vessels. While gluten-free brewing often requires longer mash times, those lag times can be solved with adding more vessels to your brew day process, breaking up the mash into two steps and even adding a whirlpool vessel to do additional flavor additions. Given certain methods in gluten-free mashing, specifically the decantation mash, you will likely need a separate vessel into which you can decant your mash liquid and cool it. At larger scales it can take quite a long time to cool hot mash liquid unless using some sort of chilling element. Most setups like these have two or more vessels, but a system that was attempting to achieve a decantation mash could require up to five different brewhouse vessels.

GELATINIZING GLUTEN-FREE GRAINS

One factor that distinguishes gluten-free brewing from conventional barley-based brewing is the higher temperatures needed to get the best out of the grain bill. To begin with, the grains that form the core of most gluten-free brewing—rice, corn (maize), millet, sorghum, and buckwheat—all have gelatinization temperatures above that of barley, so planning for higher temperatures in your process is pretty much necessary in order to get your money's worth.

Table 5.1. Gelatinization temperatures for selected brewing grains

Barley	132–143°F (56–62°C)
Buckwheat	152–165°F (67–74°C)
Corn (maize)	147–167°F (64–75°C)
Millet	147–161°F (64–72°C)
Rice	141–161°F (61–72°C)
Sorghum	160–176°F (71–80°C)
Note: Values from Ledley et al. (2021).	

Gelatinization is the first step in the solubilization and eventual enzymatic degradation of starch. Gelatinization occurs when hot water swells the grain's endosperm material, hydrating the starches to the point where the starch crystalline structure breaks apart and the individual starch chains are released. At this point the starch undergoes liquefaction, which allows enzymes like amylases and limit dextrinases to go to work on the ruptured starch molecules. In barley-based mash regimes, gelatinization takes place at temperatures in the 145–159°F (63–70°C) range, where amylases and limit dextrinases work relatively well within the thick, starchy milieu of the mash. Given the higher gelatinization temperatures required for gluten-free grains, it then follows that exogenous α-amylases that favor higher temperatures should be employed. When a brewer does not use a high-temperature α-amylase, steps should be taken to avoid denaturing endogenous amylase activity during gelatinization, specifically through the decantation method of preserving endogenous enzymes for later addition (p. 89).

Anecdotally, a higher mash resting temperature bordering on a cooking step seems necessary to extract the best attributes from grains like rice and corn, despite their gelatinization temperatures being similar to millet, sorghum, and buckwheat. Some brewers suggest that 20 minutes at 190°F (87.8°C) is a solid plan when using grains like rice and corn. For millet and buckwheat, a treatment with water that is at least 175°F (79°C) helps substantially, the higher resting temperature in conjunction with heat-stable exogenous enzymes positively improving extraction rates (Grouse Malt House, pers. comm.).

TARGETING MASH PH

Whether you plan on using endogenous or exogenous enzymes, you will need to make sure your mash pH is optimized to achieve the desired outcome. This is a best practice whether you're brewing with gluten-free grains or using barley. Most diastatic endogenous enzymes in gluten-free grains appear to have pH optima similar to their equivalents in barley, generally falling between pH 5.0 and 5.5 (Zarnkow et al. 2010, 149; Ledley et al. 2021, 9). However, bear in mind that some commercially available exogenous enzymes have optima in the pH 5.3–5.6 range, so this is important to note when planning water treatments and mash regimes in the brewhouse. As with barley mashing, you may also consider brewing salts to increase calcium ion levels to aid in achieving pH ranges closer to your target without the use of additional acids.

Given these different pH preferences, the brewer may want to start the mash at a certain pH with one enzymatic addition, then alter the pH (with additional grains or acid/base) with the introduction of another exogenous enzyme. Some brewers choose to just set pH to a range that is close enough to where the chosen enzymes work their best, very similar to how barley brewers select the appropriate conditions given the efficacy and modification level of the grains they are using. You can view gluten-free grains as similar to the needs of barley mashes that require special treatments like rising step mashes, decoction mashes, or cereal cooking steps, for example, where the barley-based grist has a high proportion of raw or unmalted grains, or the malt is less modified. In fact, the decantation mash, which takes advantage of the endogenous enzymes that are present in some gluten-free grains, is quite similar to a decoction mash method, as we will explore later in this chapter.

MASH ENZYMES IN GLUTEN-FREE BREWING

Some of the techniques that follow assume that there are not enough endogenous enzymes or high enough enzymatic activity in malted gluten-free grains to achieve the same results as would be expected when brewing with barley. Brewers that use gluten-free grains often take steps to augment the grains' endogenous enzymes with exogenous enzymes that shorten the mash rest times and speed up the brew day process generally. Some of the mash regimes that follow ignore the endogenous enzymes altogether and focus instead on adding the appropriate amount or optimal dosing rate of exogenous enzymes based on the weight of the grain bill and getting the highest efficiency possible in the shortest amount of time. Many of these exogenous enzymes mimic the enzymes that barley contains and would normally be present in a barley-based mash.

Using exogenous enzymes in gluten-free mashes does come with some considerations. For instance, the higher gelatinization temperatures many gluten-free grains require can denature the enzymes present, exogenous or endogenous. Pullulanase, which is the same class of enzyme as barley limit dextrinase, is available as an exogenous addition but does not work well above 145°F (63°C). Likewise, β-glucanase that might be found in buckwheat, for example, is denatured at a recommended higher strike temperature of 175°F (79°C), so, after an initial higher rest has been achieved that gelatinizes the starch and begins the saccharification process, additional enzyme is added once the mash falls to a lower temperature. A brewer will take such factors into account on brew day in order to make sure that brewing processes like lautering go smoothly.

Exogenous enzymes can also be combined to optimize results. Xylanases (which are a subset of pentasonases) and cellulases can degrade additional plant polysaccharides. Many brewers have specifically noticed off-flavor precursors diminishing in grains like rice when enzyme cocktails that contain enzymes like these are used, and this seems to be especially true for husky grains.

We will now explore various enzymes that can be found endogenously within some gluten-free grain kernels as well as those available from exogenous sources. As we've spoken about, there really doesn't seem to be a right or wrong way to apply these—your main focus should be the effect they have on your resulting beer. Some of these effects may be more or less desirable depending on what beer you are aiming for. For example, using enzymes that aid in mash bed drainage will make for an easier lauter but could degrade too many elements that would otherwise be desirable in the final product, like those that contribute to head retention.

DEBRANCHING ENZYMES

Limit dextrinase, commonly substituted with exogenous pullulanase, is the major debranching enzyme that helps break down the larger branched sugar chains present in the mash. Exogenous pullulanases, which function similarly to limit dextrinases in barley and millet, cleave the α-(1,6) linkages of the starch constituents amylopectin and amylose, making these starch polymers more accessible to the activity of α- and β-amylase; pullulanase also removes branch points in limit dextrins. These starches and limit dextrins are unfermentable by yeast and may provide body or sweetness in the final beer, but also contribute to undesirable hazes and off-flavors.

These debranching enzymes do much of the legwork that the endogenous enzymes in barley and other conventional brewing grains naturally do. Gelatinization is the first step to getting soluble sugars, and since most gluten-free grains need a higher temperature to gelatinize, it's almost worth treating them all like they don't have any enzymes to begin with as any that are there will not survive gelatinization.

MALTOGENIC AND GLUCOGENIC ENZYMES

Maltogenic and glucogenic enzymes in this context essentially refers to the various α-amylases that favor glucose and maltose production in the mash. Using these enzymes in concert with starch debranching enzymes during wort production is necessary with gluten-free grains to achieve a desirable degree of fermentability. These exogenous enzyme components can substantially increase the extract potential of gluten-free grains (Grouse Malt House, pers. comm.).

These maltogenic enzymes are the key to successful recipe development, allowing you to dial in your finishing gravities, which can be especially important for brewing true-to-style beers. Typically, these enzymes get used after gelatinization has already occurred, and their effectiveness (or how fermentable your wort is) is based on their contact time with the mash, mash pH, temperature, and mash thickness. Some are quite temperature stable, whereas some only work within a 5–10-degree Fahrenheit range.

It's important at this point to note that these enzymes are often referred to as saccharification enzymes, as they are the primary enzymes that break down starches to fermentable sugars. This term is commonly used to refer to β-amylase in barley brewing, but there is not a gluten-free analog in gluten-free brewing as β-amylase sources are extracted from barley. The exogenous malto- and glucogenic enzymes are achieving the same end as β-amylase, but they are not the same. So as not to confuse, we're focusing specifically on enzymes that lead to the production of glucose, maltose, and maltotriose.

Glucogenic enzymes like amyloglucosidase are commonly found in gluco-amylase exogenous enzymes and also help create fermentable glucose in the wort. Additionally, these enzymes also synthesize maltotriose in the mash. This is where getting down into the details can truly help, as specific mash treatments will lend more fermentable components, and same may throw you off when it comes to brewing to style. For example, research seems to suggest most gluten-free grains do not yield significant levels of maltotetraose (Ledley et al. 2021, 14–16), so steps like adding additional complex sugars into solution may be needed to help create the right tastes and textures in the finished beer.

USING EXOGENOUS ENZYMES

It's not cheating, it's stacking the deck in your favor.

Many exogenous enzymes commercially available contain a cocktail of enzymes like α-amylase, pullulanase (limit dextrinase), and others like β-glucanase, xylanase, lipase, and cellulase. The next section will look at specific enzyme products on the market, but table 5.2 is an overview of where in the brewing process each class of enzyme plays a role. Some aid in gelatinization and liquefaction of starches, some aid more in saccharification of the soluble starches, and some break down other components of the grains like β-glucans, fats, and proteins, among other things, to create vital yeast nutrients that would otherwise need to be added as supplements by the brewer to ensure a well-ordered fermentation. For instance, BriesSweet™ White Sorghum Extract provides only two-thirds of the necessary FAN needed by most brewer's yeast strains. The brewer will either need to add those elements or, alternatively, add other grains and the exogenous proteases that can act on those grains to make up for the FAN deficit.

Table 5.2. Stages in the brewing process and appropriate exogenous enzyme additions

Operation	Enzymes	Enzyme action	Function
Decoction vessel (cereal cooker)	α-amylase	Hydrolyse starch	Grain liquefaction* Reduce viscosity
	β-glucanase	Hydrolyse glucans	Aid the filtration
Mashing	α-amylase	Hydrolyse starch	Malt improvement
	Amyloglucosidase	Increase glucose content	Increase % fermentable sugar in "light" beer
	Debranching enzyme	Hydrolyse α-(1,6) branch points of starch	Secures maximum fermentability of the wort
	Proteases	Increase soluble protein, and free amino- nitrogen (FAN)	Malt improvement Improved yeast growth
	β-glucanase	Hydrolyse glucans	Improve wort separation
	Pentosanase/xylanase	Hydrolyse pentosans of malt, barley, wheat	Improve extraction and beer filtration
Fermentation	Fungal α-amylase	Increase maltose and glucose content	Increase % fermentable sugar in "light" beer
	β-glucanase	Hydrolyze glucans	Reduce viscosity and aid filtration
	α-acetolactate decarboxylase (ALDC)	Converts α-acetolactate to acetoin directly	Decrease fermentation time by avoiding formation of diacetyl
Conditioning tank	Protease	Modify protein-polyphenolic compounds	Reduce the chill haze formed in beer

* For starchy cereals such as maize, rice, sorghum, or pure starch materials added to the mash.

> *Gluten-free brewers don't often talk much about using exogenous β-amylases because, at this time, commercially available β-amylases are derived from barley. Recent research, for example, Ledley et al. (2021), has shown that brown and ivory teff both possess significant levels of endogenous β-amylase activity (although still less than barley). If the extraction of β-amylases from gluten-free sources such as teff can be made viable, it would mean that these enzymes could become available to brewers using gluten-free grains.*

COMMONLY AVAILABLE EXOGENOUS ENZYME BRANDS

Some of the enzymes referenced in this section are specific brand names. Many are available from online storefronts like Gluten-Free Home Brewing and Gluten-Free Brewing Supply, and usually in the size range that makes sense for a homebrewer (i.e., 4–8 fl. oz. bottles). Commercial brewers might look to companies like Novozymes® and Specialty Enzymes and Biotechnology (SEB). There are many enzyme producers out there, and you may seek out various enzyme products that mimic or possess the same active ingredients as the enzymes discussed below.

Termamyl®. A staple in the gluten-free brewing space, I would recommend Termamyl in just about any recipe, either to augment endogenous enzymes or dosed by weight of grain as if there were no endogenous enzymes. It is available in various concentrations and formulations, such as Termamyl Classic and Termamyl SC DS. Described as a "thermostable endo-acting alpha amylase," Termamyl has a wide temperature window (100–212°F, or 37–100°C) and can withstand boiling for at least 15 minutes before it denatures all the way. This enzyme is advisable for newer all-grain gluten-free brewers as well as commercial brewers since it can take just about whatever the brewhouse throws at it. The wide temperature range allows you to use Termamyl whether you are doing a rising, falling, or single-infusion mash (or really any mash regime). That said, as with any enzyme, the highest activity appears to happen toward the top end of this enzyme's temperature range, so as long as it has not denatured due to improper mash pH or extended boiling, a higher mash temperature will mean a shorter contact time is necessary, shortening the brew day.

Furthermore, if you do a longer mash, Termamyl won't transform your beer into a brut or cider, as it can produce complex sugars and maltose easily but does not appear to favor glucose production as much as other enzymes. My own trials have shown that Termamyl is a useful aid in the production of maltose, especially in rice. Termamyl SC DS seems to perform best at higher-temperature gelatinization steps with gluten-free grains like corn and rice, 190–200°F (87–93°C). These higher temperature steps help swell the starch granules, exposing more of the starch chain to the Termamyl α-amylase.

Millet and buckwheat also benefit from treatment with Termamyl SC DS, although they do not need as high of a rest temperature—175°F (79°C) seems to do just fine with grains like these (Grouse Malt House, pers. comm.). Many brewers have noted that grains like malted sorghum and oats also seem to favor these lower rest temperatures when Termamyl is in the mix (although both of these malts do have endogenous enzymes).

You can make just about any ale or lager style well using Termamyl. This enzyme does not require lengthy mash steps, as it works on contact with soluble starch in the mash and can be added to the strike water before adding in grains and malts. You will need to make sure your pH is below 6.0 to achieve this, but it can make for more consistency with brew days.

Ondea® Pro. Ondea Pro is a mixture of different enzymes consisting of α-amylase, cellulase, pullulanase, xylanase, protease, and lipase. Although this blend means Ondea Pro is easily the most expensive enzyme product listed in this chapter, and the various enzymes have differing temperatures and pH optima, it offers a lot of possibilities to the average homebrewer if they can obtain it. That said, it is important to disclaim that you need specific brewhouse abilities to truly get your money's worth out of this product. Ondea Pro was originally concocted as a solution for traditional brewhouses using high-adjunct grists and raw or unmalted barley, due to the blend's ability to extract sugars out of such grains without using a cereal cooking step. You will still need to do a gelatinization step to be most successful with grains like rice and corn, but you can accomplish this through a slow rising step mash, which usually takes around 2 hours and 45 minutes all said and done. If you omit a lower temperature rest in the 114–130°F (46–54°C) range, you will denature the more heat-sensitive enzymes, in effect limiting the protease, cellulase, and xylanase components from doing their work. These lower temperature rests help ensure good levels of FAN and soluble peptides for foam stability. These enzymes also contribute to an easy lauter, which can help you reduce time taken and the cost of additional ingredients like rice hulls.

Grains like rice have shown much more promise when using enzyme cocktails like Ondea Pro. While a useful source of fermentables and soluble nitrogen, rice can act against the presence of other desirable qualities in finished beer, noticeably lasting foam. Rice contains a relatively high fat content by weight, the bulk of these lipids being present in the husk. Lipids, being hydrophobic ("water hating") destabilize foam. Incorporating Ondea Pro into your mash offers a way for you to brew all-grain recipes with significant quantities of rice where a cereal cook is not possible and still produce a beer that displays prominent and residual foam and lacing down the glass.

The longer mash period with Ondea Pro has been shown to be foolproof, but some brewers may be able to reduce this time, if needed; specifically, with smaller grain bills at the homebrew scale or pilot scale, the full 2 hour and 45 minutes might not be absolutely necessary. In fact, the potency that many brewers speak of when referring to Ondea Pro motivated me to experiment with shorter rest times. I have produced good yields of fermentable wort (i.e., some of the highest levels of glucose, maltose, and maltotriose) with Ondea Pro and Ceremix® Flex mash regimes taking 1 hour and 20 minutes; thus, at a small batch or homebrew level, shortened rest times can still achieve similarly high efficiencies. This is an area where I would welcome brewers to share their results as this will help inform best practices.

Many brewers that have used just Ondea Pro have noted higher finishing gravities, so, while this enzyme cocktail does possess α-amylase, it seems to benefit from being paired with other enzymes like Ceremix Flex or Termamyl (or both), as these are more temperature-stable α-amylases.

Ondea Pro has opened up new opportunities for gluten-free brewers because of its notable improvements to extract potentials; this is the main reason it caught on in gluten-free brewing, especially where cereal cooking just isn't an option in the brewhouse. Grains like rice that would typically be estimated to yield 20–25 PPG (167–209 l°/kg) are now weighing in at 30–35 PPG (250–292 l°/kg) This massive increase in efficiency immediately changes how many brewers formulate recipes or how gluten-free recipe kits are built. What can make a huge difference is the reduction in grains needed for the resulting beer, helping bring the overall cost of making the beer down, which is a huge consideration for commercial brewers but also homebrewers who generally have to pay more by weight for gluten-free grains than their barley equivalents.

SEBAmyl® L. A fungal derived maltogenic α-amylase, SEBAmyl L works best between 140°F and 160°F (60–71°C); performance diminishes from there, with the enzyme denaturing completely at 168°F (75°C). Typically used in concert with SEBAmyl BAL 100 or Termamyl, SEBAmyl L can also be used with products like Ondea Pro. SEBAmyl L has been featured in gluten-free recipes for nearly a decade at this point. When used at 1.0–1.5 mL per pound of malt (2.2–3.3 mL/kg), this enzyme delivers good maltose and glucose extraction. Having tried various mash regimes featuring SEBAmyl L, I have found that mashes treated with SEBAmyl L in conjunction with Termamyl, both rising and falling step mashes, can achieve extraction efficiencies of 100% or more for both malted millet from Grouse and malted rice from Eckert. In a mixed mash of millet, rice, and buckwheat, efficiency was 99.5% in a falling step mash.

Although many brewers have also used SEBAmyl L in single-infusion mashes, its best performance comes when all available starches are soluble and it needs to be added to the mash after gelatinization has already occurred, which means that it is best employed in a step mash.

SEBAmyl® BAL 100. SEBAmyl BAL 100 is a bacterially derived α-amylase that produces dextrins and works well between 140°F and 168°F (60–76°C), denaturing above 168°F. This enzyme is not as widely used nowadays, as many brewers have noticed much higher extract efficiencies when using more temperature-stable enzymes.

Saczyme® Pro 1.5X. Saczyme Pro 1.5X is a fast-acting amyloglucosidase that works best between 150°F and 155°F (66–68°C). Its fast action means it is more commonly known as an enzyme for brewers who will be distilling the resulting beer into a spirit, and it only needs about 30 minutes of contact time to produce highly fermentable wort that yields more alcohol. Your hot sparge water will denature it quickly and allow you to dial in your wort profile.

While popular for distilling, further research is needed to truly understand how Saczyme Pro 1.5X can best be used for brewing. Drier styles like light lagers, Belgian wits, saisons, certain IPAs (like brut IPA, for instance) might benefit from the type of highly fermentable wort that an enzyme like this can produce. Even a Belgian tripel might benefit from a recipe that employs Saczyme Pro 1.5X due to the higher levels of glucose that it produces with normal contact times—as discussed in chapter 4, some degree of stress may be ideal for styles like tripel fermented with Belgian ale yeast.

Ultimase® BWL 40. Ultimase BWL 40 is an enzyme cocktail used primarily for viscosity reduction, as it is a blend of β-glucanase and xylanase that aids in β-glucan and xylan hydrolysis in the mash. This is a specific consideration for certain grain bills containing pseudocereals like quinoa and malted or unmalted buckwheat.

Fungamyl® BrewQ. As its name suggests, Fungamyl BrewQ is another maltogenic α-amylase derived from a fungal species. This product is great for extracting maltose and glucose. Fungamyl BrewQ works best around 140–160°F (60–71°C). The more you use, the more fermentable the wort is, so you can work to dial in your finishing gravity based on your dosing rate. Further research is needed with this enzyme to formulate best uses for brewing gluten-free true-to-style beers.

Fungamyl BrewQ enzyme is also used in commercial bread baking, where it helps with consistency among varied flour mixes.

Ceremix® Flex. Ceremix Flex is another product that does away with the need for a cereal cooking step. In gluten-free brewing, Ceremix Flex is most commonly used with Ondea Pro, but Termamyl is also an option. Ceremix Flex is a maltogenic enzyme blend, consisting of α-amylase and pullulanase and is designed to be used by itself. From my experience, and the experience of others in forums like the Zero Tolerance Gluten-Free Homebrew Club, best results with this product seem to come after gelatinization or in concert with enzymes that aid in starch degradation. The best temperature range for Ceremix Flex appears to be 145–180°F (63–82°C).

As also reported by many brewers using the Zero Tolerance forum, an additional benefit to using Ceremix Flex is that single-infusion mashes work well: a 45 to 90-minute rest at 170–180°F (76–82°C) seems to yield consistent results in terms of sugar extraction, which helps simplify the brewing process with gluten-free grains. In my own experiments, single-infusion mashes performed with just Ceremix Flex on malted millet and malted rice resulted in 99.9% extract efficiencies for both, based on the assumed extract potentials for those malts. Trials I did with other enzyme and mash regimes returned higher than 100% efficiencies but the single-infusion method is, of course, much simpler. For those brewers that can only do single-infusion mashing, the fact that Ceremix Flex can achieve these results is noteworthy.

AMG® 300 L BrewQ. AMG 300 L BrewQ is an amyloglucosidase that is seemingly good for producing high levels of maltose and glucose, based on dramatic increases seen in gluten-free wort fermentability that result in 87%–97% apparent attenuation in millet and millet/buckwheat mashes when used in conjunction with Termamyl (Grouse Malt House, pers. comm.). AMG300 L BrewQ has even been used by some brewers to aid in stuck fermentations, although this is not recommended unless the brewer has the ability to denature the enzyme, a task usually done in commercial breweries through pasteurization.[1]

Attenuzyme® Core. Attenuzyme Core is a powerful amyloglucosidase (a.k.a. glucoamylase) that acts on dextrins and maltotriose to increase the proportion of glucose in the wort. Using Attenuzyme will increase the degree of attenuation, drying out a beer. To control how dry the beer will finish, you must control the enzyme's contact time with the wort. One useful practice that allows more control over this process is dosing a portion of the wort separately and limiting contact time to 30 minutes. This method has led to predictable results. It is vital that the portion of wort dosed with Attenuzyme be added to boiling wort to instantly denature the enzyme.

Using Attenuzyme Core: At the end of the mash, collect the first third of the mash runnings into a separate bucket and set this aside. You can send the remaining two-thirds of the runnings to the kettle and start heating it in preparation for the boil. When you are 30 minutes away from reaching the boil, dose the set aside mash runnings with Attenuzyme Core at a

---

[1] A stuck fermentation can happen for a couple of reasons, such as yeast health, quantities of soluble fermentable sugars, and the specific yeast strain; for example, if you produce high quantities of unfermentable sugars in your mash. Unsticking a stuck fermentation usually involves pitching additional yeast, pitching a different yeast strain, or adding additional yeast nutrients and energizers to the fermentor. However, using an enzyme to degrade complex sugars in the fermenting liquid should, in theory, aid in creating more fermentable glucose and maltose that the stalled yeast can then use.

rate of 1 mL/lb. grist (2.2 mL/kg). After allowing 30 minutes of contact time with the enzyme, the dosed mash portion is added to the boiling wort, denaturing the enzyme. This process increases the fermentability of the wort, leading to finishing gravities below 1.010 SG (2.6°P). Attenuzyme Core can break down the complex sugars produced in the original mash with enzymes like Ondea Pro and Ceremix Flex.

Powdered α-amylase. If the specialist enzyme products already described are not easy to find, α-amylase powders can be a great option to use in the mash, assuming you have made all of the starches soluble. You won't be able to get many dextrins into solution, however, so you will want to use grains that possess endogenous limit dextrinase in order to extract them if desired in the final beer. In theory, a rising step mash or falling step mash could be used with this enzyme, but the temperature range may vary depending on the brand, and many denature above 170°F (76°C). **You must also check the brand you use is gluten free**, as not all of them are.

MASH METHODS

As discussed in chapter 4, the best renditions of gluten-free recipes will likely feature a couple of different types of grain and pseudocereal, many of which have drastically different gelatinization temperatures and enzymatic activities. Many of the following mash regimes seek to rectify these differences, or to compensate for certain things that the grains may lack. Some of these methods are more applicable to specific ingredients. For example, buckwheat and quinoa favor protein and β-glucan rests (p. 51), while rice and corn benefit from a higher rest temperature north of 180°F (82°C).

Remember, there is no right or wrong way, but the goal is to focus on producing wort with the specific profile of sugars (fermentable and unfermentable), proteins, and yeast nutrients in solution so that you can make the best true-to-style beer possible. Even if you have some noticeable limitations facing you, you will be able to make amazing gluten-free beer.

DECANTATION METHOD

The decantation method of mashing can be thought of as a modified decoction mash. There are several variations on the decantation mash, some being modified versions of similar processes used in barley mashing (Ledley et al. 2021, 6). A popular and effective method used by gluten-free homebrewers is commonly known as the "Lavery method" (https://glutenfreehomebrewing .com/tutorials.php) and will be the method focused on here. The process involves a lower mash-in temperature to do a protein and/or β-glucan rest; during this rest, the endogenous enzymes are pulled out from the crushed grains and into solution in the mash. Once these enzymes are in solution, typically after 25 minutes at rest temperature, about two-thirds of the mash liquid is separated from the mash and held to one side, and oftentimes cooled. Meanwhile, the remainder of the mash is heated to nearly boiling temperatures to gelatinize the grains and then allowed to start to cool down. The cooler decanted liquid is reintroduced to the wort when the wort has cooled down to around 158°F (70°C), which should bring the mash temperature into the optimal range for saccharification and avoids overdiluting the mash or denaturing the enzymes.

This decantation method is suggested for those that don't have access to exogenous enzymes, as this method requires some extra steps and a thinner mash because of the multiple rising and falling temperature steps. Always be cognizant of the fact that the gelatinization point of the gluten-free grains you're employing is higher than the denaturing point of their endogenous α-amylases. Without the decanted enzyme-rich solution, you will not be able to convert the starches in your mash. This method would be nearly impossible to use on a commercial scale without a specially designed facility.

The decantation method can be thought of as a modified decoction mash because it involves part of the mash being separated and then recombined, but there are obviously key differences. For instance, a decoction mash involves boiling a small part of the mash grains for starch degradation, while in a decantation mash the whole of the grain portion is subjected to near-boiling temperatures while the enzyme-laden brewing liquid is temporarily separated from the mash.

DECANTATION MASH STEP BY STEP

The steps to perform a mash using the decantation method are as follows:

Instructions are for a 4.5 US gal. (17 L) recipe batch.

1. Mash into 2 gal. (7.6 L) strike water at 109°F (42.7°C).
   - Hold for β-glucan rest at 104°F (40°C) for 25 minutes, stirring every 10 minutes.
   - Make sure the mash pH is at 5.4 (use citric, phosphoric, or lactic acid to adjust).
2. Add 0.8 gal. (3.0 L) of boiling water.
   - Hold for protein rest at 131°F (55°C) for 25 min; allow to settle for the last 15 minutes.
3. Decant off 1 gal. (3.8 L) of clear wort from the top and refrigerate.
4. Infuse 0.5 gal. (1.9 L) of boiling water into mash.
   - Heat mash to 158°F (70°C) for partial conversion; hold for 20 minutes.
5. Bring mash to a boil and hold for 5 minutes. Depending on your heat source, you may need to stir often to avoid scorching the grains onto the bottom of the kettle.
6. Cool mash back to 158°F (70°C).
7. Add the decanted liquid to achieve a mash temperature of 149°F (65°C).
   - Hold for saccharification rest for 90 minutes.
8. Sparge and boil as usual.

Employing the decantation method requires no exogenous enzymes, but you will need to use a grain bill that features malted millet or malted sorghum as your base grain for their endogenous α-amylase and limit dextrinase activity, malted buckwheat for its β-amylase contribution, and pregelatinized rice malt for available sugars that those enzymes can work on. Millet itself has a much higher limit dextrinase activity (around 500 U/kg at optimal pH of 5.2) than any other commonly available gluten-free grain, and helps ensure you achieve higher extract potential (Ledley 2021, 9). My own experiments using the decantation mash on Grouse's pale millet malt resulted in an extract yield somewhere around 33 PPG (275 l°/kg), over 100% efficiency if you consider the expected extract potential for this malt is 29 PPG (242 l°/kg). That same decantation mash trial showed glucose, maltose, and maltotriose levels in the resulting wort commensurate with those worts produced using exogenous enzymes. Zarnkow et al. (2010, 149) and Ledley et al. (2021, 15) also showed that the levels of fermentable sugars from mashed millet are similar to those from barley, and only seem to be lacking maltotetraose. This is another factor that seems to explain the relatively higher finishing gravities that barley beers experience compared with gluten-free beers, as results from the decantation method seem to suggest that gluten-free grains and malts contribute mostly fermentable sugars to a wort.

TRADITIONAL GLUTEN-FREE MASH METHODS

Traditional millet and sorghum beer brewers across Africa don't really care about enzymes nor have trouble fermenting the wort, so don't worry too much if you do not have exogenous enzymes to fall back on. The longer, often overnight, mashes employed in these millet or sorghum beers rely on the grains' endogenous enzymes to create a fermentable wort, as well as some other helpful friends, like bacteria.

Recent research, such as Zarnkow et al. (2010) and Ledley et al. (2021), demonstrates the validity of traditional brewers' methods. Millet exhibits some intrinsic β-amylase and α-amylase activity, albeit much lower than found in barley, and significant levels of intrinsic limit dextrinase activity; sorghum likewise displays low levels of β-amylase activity and moderate levels of α-amylase and limit dextrinase activity (Zarnkow et al. 2010, 142; Ledley et al. 2021, 9). These attributes would create a somewhat fermentable wort with relatively higher levels of dextrins in solution. In traditional brewing, the microflora present on the grains would lend their endogenous enzymes as well, thus, the traditional method of overnight mashing would then help create a more fermentable wort in addition to lowering the pH.

SINGLE-INFUSION MASH

A recipe that employs a single-infusion mash should focus on using grains that gelatinize within or close to the desired rest range, like millet and buckwheat for example. This mash regime can, in theory, be pulled off with an enzyme blend product. Ceremix Flex, for example, can potentially be used by itself when employing a single-infusion mash. Use Termamyl SC DS, Ceremix Flex, or some combination thereof, and you will likely achieve an amazing product. The temperature stability that the two of these enzymes provide will allow for a higher rest temperature and good extraction.

> Many single-infusion mash brewers avoid using more than 5%–10% malted rice or corn in recipes that don't go above 170°F (77°C) because the efficiency is too low otherwise. In cases like this, such malts are best used as character malts or adjuncts in mash regimes where the temperature will not get to the temperature at which the grains will fully gelatinize. Grains like millet, sorghum, oats, and buckwheat might be a better choice in these types of recipes.

Single Infusion with Ceremix Flex

- Mash in with strike water at 186°F (86°C), adding water treatment salts and Ceremix Flex once one-third of the grain has been added. Use the recommended dosing rate of 1 mL enzyme per pound of grain in the mash (2.2 mL/kg) for the Ceremix Flex. Rest at 170°F (76°C) for 45–90 minutes.

Alternate Low-Temperature Single Infusion Mash

- Mash in with strike water at 160°F (71°C), adding Ceremix Flex once one-third of the grain has been added. Use the recommended dosing rate of 1 mL enzyme per pound of grain in the mash (2.2 mL/kg) for the Ceremix Flex. Rest at 145°F (63°C) for 60–120 minutes.
- For the last 30 minutes of the mash, add one of the following to pull additional fermentable sugars into solution: Ondea Pro, Termamyl SC DS, or Saczyme Pro 1.5X. Start with a dosing rate of 1 mL/lb. of grain (2.2 mL/kg).

STEP MASHES

Step mashes are seen as the gluten-free brewing industry best practice, whether you use a falling temperature mash regime (from high to low temperatures) or a rising temperature mash regime (low to high). Regardless of the system you have available or your enzymes of choice, step mashing is the tried-and-true method that will allow you to produce great wort even when you're using high quantities of unmodified gluten-free grains. Two-, three-, and four-step mashes all have their place, depending on what enzymes you are looking to activate in conjunction with the grain bill to achieve specific flavors and styles effectively.

Falling temperature step mash. The falling temperature step mash regime is one of the best ways to be able to use any gluten-free grain available to you, especially unmalted grains, which already possess very low enzymatic activity but can contribute great beer-making compounds. The method involves a high strike temperature to ensure gelatinization and the addition of a thermostable α-amylase in the beginning to start the process of breaking down starches to fermentable sugars. The mash is then cooled to the saccharification enzymes' temperature optimum. This optimal second temperature rest can be achieved by adding the grains that gelatinize at lower temperatures, with the heat capacity of these cooler grains reducing the temperature of the mash liquid; and, if the grains are not enough, you can also add some cold water to bring the temperature down (similar to how it's done with the decantation method).

Since there is typically not a protein rest in this process, viscosity-reducing enzymes will be a huge factor in promoting a successful brew day, as they take the place of the lower-temperature protein and β-glucan rests. Yes, there are some trade-offs with this mash regime; for instance, only certain, specific thermostable α-amylases like Termamyl SC DS can be considered. Before products like Ondea Pro and Ceremix Flex came out, the falling temperature step mash regime was seen as the best way (if not the only way) to get 95% efficiency and above, and many gluten-free brewers still swear by it.

Despite the efficacy of the falling temperature step mash, only a minority of gluten-free homebrewers currently employ this method. It is much more common at the commercial level, because this method represents the best throughput.

A falling temperature step mash can be done in several ways, four examples of which follow here. These procedures are for brewing a regular homebrew batch of five gallons (18.9 L):

Falling Temperature Step Mash with Single Mash-In: Millet and Buckwheat
Use this procedure if your grain bill uses only millet or millet and buckwheat as base malts.
1. Heat 5 gal. (18.9 L) strike water to 186°F (86°C) and mash in, adding water treatment salts and Termamyl SC DS once one-third of the grain has been added. Use the recommended dosing rate of 1 mL enzyme per pound of grain in the mash (2.2 mL/kg).
2. Rest at 170°F (76°C) for 30 minutes.
3. Add 1 gal. (3.8 L) room-temperature or cold water; the mash temperature should go down to or below 160°F (71°C) at this point. Vorlauf until temperature is reached, if necessary.
4. Once below 160°F (71°C), add AMG 300 L BrewQ at 1.25 mL/lb. of grain (2.75 mL/kg) to create additional fermentable sugars and help with mash viscosity.

Falling Temperature Step Mash with Single Mash-In: Rice, Corn, Unmalted Grain
Use this procedure if your grain bill contains rice, corn, or any unmalted grains.
1. Heat 5 gal. (18.9 L) strike water to 205°F (96°C) and mash in, adding water treatment salts and Termamyl SC DS once one-third of the grain has been added. Use the recommended dosing rate of 1 mL enzyme per pound of grain in the mash (2.2 mL/kg).
2. Rest at 190°F (87°C) for 30 minutes.
3. Add 1.0–1.5 gal. (3.8–5.7 L) room-temperature or cold water; the mash temperature should go down to or below 160°F (71°C) at this point. Vorlauf until temperature is reached, if necessary.
4. Once below 160°F (71°C), add AMG 300 L BrewQ at 1.25 mL/lb. of grain (2.75 mL/kg) to create additional fermentable sugars and help with mash viscosity.

The next two procedures involve multiple mash-in stages to account for corn and rice, which have high gelatinization temperatures. One additional benefit of doing a separate high-temperature rest with these grains is that they will be mixed with the high-temperature α-amylase immediately, which can reduce the time needed in later rests since these enzymes have already begun to do their job even as the starch molecules are swelling during gelatinization.

Falling Temperature Step Mash with Multiple Mash-Ins: 50% Rice

Use this procedure if your grain bill consists of 50% rice malt and 50% lower-gelatinization-temperature grains (millet, buckwheat, oats, etc.).

1. Heat 2.5 gal. (9.5 L) strike water to 205°F (96°C). Mash in with the rice malt only, adding Termamyl SC DS once one-third of the rice malt has been added. Use the recommended dosing rate of 1 mL enzyme per pound of grain in the mash (2.2 mL/kg).
2. Rest for 20 minutes at 190°F (88°C).
3. Once this rest is completed, stir in the remainder of your lower-gelatinization-temperature grains. Add 2.5 gal. (9.5 L) room-temperature or cold water as the mash gets thicker and harder to stir; the mash temperature should be at or below 160°F (71°C) at this point. Vorlauf until temperature is reached, if necessary.
4. Once below 160°F (71°C), add AMG 300 L BrewQ at 1.25 mL/lb. of grain (2.75 mL/kg) to create additional fermentable sugars and help with mash viscosity.

Falling Temperature Step Mash with Multiple Mash-Ins: 50% Corn

Use this procedure if your grain bill consists of 50% corn malt and 50% lower-gelatinization-temperature grains (millet, buckwheat, oats, etc.).

1. Heat 2.5 gal. (9.5 L) strike water to boiling, 212°F (100°C). Mash in with the corn malt only, adding Termamyl SC DS once one-third of the corn malt has been added. Use the recommended dosing rate of 1 mL enzyme per pound of grain in the mash (2.2 mL/kg).
2. Rest for 30 minutes at 200°F (93°C).
3. Once this rest is completed, stir in the remainder of your lower-gelatinization-temperature grains. Add 2.5 gal. (9.5 L) room-temperature or cold water as the mash gets thicker and harder to stir; the mash temperature should be at or below 160°F (71°C) at this point. Vorlauf until temperature is reached, if necessary.
4. Once below 160°F (71°C), add AMG 300 L BrewQ at 1.25 mL/lb. of grain (2.75 mL/kg) to create additional fermentable sugars and help with mash viscosity.

Regardless of your step mash procedure, it is always smart to vorlauf until your wort passes the iodine test to show conversion is complete (the timing of this will vary based on your setup). From there, you can sparge and boil. Since temperature is not as much of a concern when mash pH is dialed in, sparging with near boiling water won't really hurt anything. If the mash bed is set up from your vorlauf, and as long as the flow rate is dialed in, you should be in a great position to avoid channeling and loss of efficiency. This falling temperature mash method could be pulled off with Termamyl SC DS and Ceremix Flex, but can also be done with Termamyl SC DS in conjunction with AMG 300 L BrewQ, Fungamyl BrewQ, SebAmyl L, and Saczyme Pro 1.5X.

Some products don't make sense for a falling mash regime; specifically, Ondea Pro—mashing in anywhere above 140°F (60°C) denatures most of the enzymes that make this enzyme blend so special.

Rising temperature step mash. The rising temperature step mash regime is the most common brewing method among gluten-free homebrewers. Ondea Pro and Ceremix Flex are currently the most popular enzyme cocktail, but previous to these enzymes being widely available, a rising temperature step mash regime was achieved with other enzymes, such as Termamyl and SEBAmyl L. It can even be done with powdered α-amylase, just make sure it's from a reliable gluten-free source. The goal is to add to the endogenous enzymes with exogenous enzymes.

Rising step mashes are particularly popular because they employ a β-glucan rest (typically 118–135°F, or 48–57°C). This is basically what allows you to avoid a sludge on top of your filter bed that can develop when you vorlauf with uncoverted starches present in the mash, and these rests can help create a nice pillowy mash all on its own.

Rising Temperature Step Mash: Suggested Best Practice
1. Mash in at 125°F (52°C) for a 30-minute β-glucan rest.
2. After the β-glucan rest, you can take two routes depending on how fast your system heats. You will need to throttle back when using a heating element like a propane burner, as those heat the mash faster than electric systems, and you may denature too many enzymes too fast to achieve the correct extraction.
   a. If your system is capable of rapidly heating the mash, you can break out the temperature rise into three discrete 30-minute rests: 145°F (63°C), 165°F (74°C), and 180°F (82°C). However, you may also need to stir consistently to ensure the enzymes are not denatured prematurely, which could be counterproductive when trying to set up your mash bed.
   b. For slower heating systems, a slow rise to 175°F (79°C) can take one and a half hours. If your system takes some time to raise the temperature, the enzymes will still do what they need to as your mash slowly rises through the various temperature ranges, and this can be an ideal method.
3. Once you are at 180°F (82°C), rest for up to 30 minutes (especially if you are using rice as a base malt), then sparge and boil.

Remember, the goal is to make sure the yeast is happy, and stressed fermentations from worts high in simple sugars are common for newer brewers who are still dialing in their process (you may want to start with certain styles like Belgian beers to get the most out of your early experiences). For ingredients like rice or corn, off-flavors typically develop when the yeast does not have enough nutrients, for instance, due to lack of FAN because proteins are poorly solubilized by enzyme activity. Having supplementary yeast nutrients on hand is a good fail-safe, and many brewers just add them as a precaution even though it may not always be necessary.

SEBAmyl L and Termamyl SC DS: Rising temperature step mash. The recommended dosing rate is 1mL per pound of grain in the mash for Termamyl (2.2 mL/kg) and 1.5 mL per pound with SEBAmyl L (3.3 mL/kg).

The important first step involves strike water with salts and enzymes added at 118–135°F (48–57°C) for a β-glucan rest lasting up to 30 minutes. From this point, you will do two successive temperature raises: one that is in the optimal temperature range for SEBamyl L (150–155°F, or 66–68°C), and one that is in the optimal temperature range for Termamyl SC DS and gelatinization, with 170–180°F (77–82°C) being the gelatinization temperature for malted millet and 190°F (88°C) for rice. Termamyl SC DS comes into its own here because of its thermostability, being able to degrade starch at just about any temperature your mash moves through during the mash steps; it just might need a little bit more contact time since it will not be operating in its optimal temperature range. These enzymes working in conjunction with the endogenous limit dextrinase of a grain like millet really helps in getting high efficiency in the mash.

Approaching this in a homebrew setting could look something like this:
1. After the β-glucan/protein rest, raise the temperature to 155°F (68°C) for a 30–60-minute saccharification rest.
2. Raise the temperature to 175°F (79°C) for a 30-minute rest. This step is to help pull out any additional starches and cleave them before separating the mash from the wort.
3. Sparge and boil. Since your second rest temperature is already high, you can sparge/lauter with water that is 180°F (82°C) all the way to boiling. In fact, you can in theory sparge with boiling water whenever a thermostable enzyme like Termamyl is used. One additional benefit of this is that there is typically a shorter time to boil since your collected liquid in the boil kettle is already hotter.

Ondea Pro and Ceremix Flex: Rising temperature step mash. The recommended dosing rate is 1mL per pound of grain in the mash of each enzyme cocktail (2.2 mL/kg).

A lower temperature rest seems to be ideal for the pullulanase, cellulase, xylanase, protease, and lipase enzymes in Ondea Pro to help create soluble protein peptides for more body and foam stability as well as to produce FAN for yeast nutrition. The α-amylases and pullulanases in both Ondea Pro and Ceremix Flex together work to provide a mix of complex sugars and fermentable sugars that can be useful when brewing many beer styles.

Thinking about the bigger picture, it makes sense to use enzymes that don't provide too much redundancy in your mash. The pullulanases within Ondea Pro and Ceremix Flex are great in a grain containing a large proportion of rice, but in concert with millet's endogenous limit dextrinase the pullulanase may, in fact, be redundant. My own experiments comparing this enzyme treatment with the decantation mash using pale millet malt (p. 89) seem to support this conjecture. It is something that warrants further research.

Whichever method you use, once your mash is complete, you will have a sweet wort rich in fermentables and nutrients for your yeast to ferment. While your brewing system will have certain limitations one way or the other, the many different choices of mash regime and enzymatic components means you do not have to be concerned that your system cannot produce great gluten-free beers. Any brewer can accomplish gluten-free beers on their system given the right conditions.

Once your wort is collected into the boil kettle, where you go from there depends entirely on the style of beer you're pursuing. Your hopping rates will vary drastically depending on the gravity of the wort in the boil, just the same as with barley brewing. Yeast pitching rates are likewise similarly influenced by the gravity of your wort, but some grains will need additional yeast nutrients even if malted versions are used (like sorghum, corn, and rice) whereas others may not (like millet, buckwheat, and quinoa). Some yeasts may avoid more complex sugars, so be on the lookout for enzyme cocktails that will create the correct precursors in your wort for the yeast you intend to use. Brewers who consistently find their finishing gravities are low will need to make changes to their mash regime and enzyme cocktail if they wish to brew styles like sweet stouts or other styles that call for higher finishing gravities. Whether you are entering into a competition or not, what you call a beer is important style-wise, as those flavors are guided by a rich brewing tradition in barley and are just as achievable with gluten-free grains.

Many of these considerations are included in the recipe chapters that follow in the second half of this book. All the beer recipes presented take these factors into account and have produced world-class beers, and some have medals to prove it. Happy brewing!

English Bitter | © Getty/mikedabell

6

British and Irish Styles

ost famous for their ales, Britain and Ireland have produced many beer styles with some incredible tastes and flavors, from light to dark, from malty to hoppy, from balanced to boozy. There is a certain amount of lore surrounding these beer styles, but do not let the debates over brewing history put you off—they have been some of the main influences for the modern craft beer scene. From being the home of the original India pale ale, porter, and stout, the British Isles has some of the most ephemeral mystique of any place in the world of beer.

Gluten-free grains can make some amazing renditions of these beer styles, and some of the recipes that follow have won awards. Let's explore!

HOOLIGAN'S ENGLISH BITTER
Gluten-Free English Bitter

Contributed by Beliveau Farm

Following the successful founding of a bed and breakfast and then a winery, Yvan and Joyce Beliveau decided to add a brewery. Yvan has a gluten intolerance and was interested in offering a gluten-free beer on tap. Yvan connected with John Hildreth, who had been researching and brewing gluten-free beer for several years. After a few conversations and curated tastings, Yvan and Joyce were so taken with the quality of John's beers that they

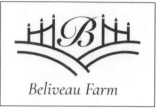

decided to go all-in with a dedicated gluten-free brewery with John as head brewer. John's goal is to use grains such as malted rice, millet, and buckwheat to create delicious and flavorful beer that is indistinguishable from that made with barley malt.

This recipe started out as one of John's most popular homebrews, and is named for his British expat friend J.D., who is a total soccer hooligan. During John's first few years of gluten-free brewing research and development, friends throughout the community were trying his beers and providing feedback, and the Hooligan's English Bitter was consistently loved and requested. It is a staple on tap at Beliveau Farm and regularly asked for by customers. Below is a five-gallon, all-grain homebrew version.

For 5 US gal. (18.9 L)

Original gravity: 1.050 SG (12.4°P)
Final gravity: 1.010–1.015 (2.6–3.8°P)
Color: 7.6 SRM (15 EBC)

IBU: 40
ABV: 4.6%–5.3%

FERMENTABLES
3.5 lb. (1.59 kg) Grouse pale millet malt*
2.5 lb. (1.13 kg) Eckert pale rice malt*
2.0 lb. (0.91 kg) Eckert biscuit rice malt 4°L
1.0 lb. (0.45 kg) Eckert crystal rice

1.0 lb. (0.45 kg) Grouse caramel millet 4°L
0.6 lb. (0.27 kg) Grouse roasted malted buckwheat
0.6 lb. (0.27 kg) Grouse pale buckwheat malt

ENZYMES
11 mL Ceremix® Flex
11 mL Ondea® Pro
11 mL Termamyl®

WATER
7.6 gal. (28.77 L) distilled water (important for mash pH)
1 tbsp + ½ tsp (9 g) gypsum
1¾ tsp (4.5 g) calcium chloride
1½ tsp (7.3 mL) lactic acid (88% solution)

HOPS
2.0 oz. (57 g) East Kent Golding (4%–6% AA) @ 60 min.
0.6 oz. (17 g) Fuggle (2.5%–6% AA) @ 10 min.

ADDITIONAL INGREDIENTS
4.00 oz. (0.11 kg) tapioca maltodextrin (to be added during boil as a slurry)
0.15 oz. (4.3 g) Irish moss @ 10 min.

YEAST
1 sachet (11.5 g, or 0.4 oz.) SafAle™ S-04 English Ale yeast

BREWING NOTES
1. Use 3.47 gal. (13.14 L) of the water for strike water and reserve the remaining for your fly or batch sparge.
2. Rising-step mash part one: Heat strike water to 135–140°F (57–60°C) and add gypsum and calcium chloride, stirring to dissolve. Add milled grains and stir to mix and evenly distribute rice hulls from the rice malts. Add all three enzymes and the lactic acid.
3. After the mash-in, the mash temperature will be around 130–134°F (54–57°C); mash pH should come in at 5.2–5.3. Mash for 45 minutes, gradually raising the temperature to and holding it at 145°F (63°C).
4. While the rising-step mash is underway, make a maltodextrin slurry. While mashing proceeds, the maltodextrin should dissolve in the water. Stir if needed.
5. Rising-step mash part two: gradually raise mash temperature to 164°F (73°C) over 45 minutes (you can go as high as 170°F, or 77°C). When finished, hold for an additional 15 minutes.
6. Before the mash is finished, preheat sparge water to 180°F (82°C). At the end of the mash, perform your sparge to collect a pre-boil volume of approximately 6 gal. (22.7 L).
7. Add the maltodextrin slurry to the wort and stir to mix in before the beginning of the boil.
8. When the boil is complete, cool the wort and transfer to the fermentor. Pitch yeast and ferment at 64°F (18°C) until specific gravity is stable and fermentation is complete. Rack to a secondary fermentor and let sit for another week.
9. Bottle when ready, allowing two weeks for bottle conditioning before drinking. If kegging, allow the requisite time needed for carbonation to equilibrate. Carbonate to 2.3 vol. CO_2.

ADDITIONAL NOTES
* If you are doing brew-in-a-bag (BIAB), you will want to slightly increase your enzyme dosage and add an extra few pounds of pale malt to your grain bill. So, fermentables will include 5 lb. (2.27 kg) of pale millet malt and 3.5 lb. (1.59 kg) of pale rice malt, and use 18 mL each of Ceremix Flex, Ondea Pro, and Termamyl.

DARK AND MILD

Gluten-Free Dark Mild

Contributed by Robert Keifer

When it comes to drinking beer, dark mild has got to be one of my favorites, not only for its ses-sionability, but for its incredible balance. Notes of toast, caramel, pumpernickel bread, and sometimes anise and maple, these are playful and inviting, with a smooth texture and clean finish. I cannot say enough good things about this style and had to make sure this recipe got into the book. The recipe here employs a rising step mash with multiple mash-in steps, which involves mashing the rice alone first with the thermostable enzyme at a hotter temperature. However, if this mash regime does not make sense for you, you can achieve this style with any other mash regime suitable for gluten-free grains.

For 5 US gal. (18.9 L)

Original gravity: 1.047 (11.7°P) **IBU:** 15
Final gravity: 1.011 (2.8°P) **ABV:** 4.7%
Color: 45 SRM (89 EBC)

FERMENTABLES

1.0 lb. (0.45 kg) Eckert biscuit rice malt 15°L
0.5 lb. (0.23 kg) Eckert biscuit rice malt 18°L
4 oz. (113 g) Eckert Pitch Black rice malt

4.5 lb. (2.04 kg) Grouse pale millet malt
1.0 lb. (0.45 kg) Grouse Goldfinch Millet malt
1.0 lb. (0.45 kg) Grouse raw millet

ENZYMES

8.25 mL Termamyl® SC DS (equivalent to 1.0 mL/lb. grain, or 2.2 mL/kg)
14.85 mL Ceremix® Flex (1.8 mL/lb., or 3.97 mL/kg)
9.9 mL Ondea® Pro (1.2 mL/lb., or 2.65 mL/kg)

WATER

Aim for a "Manchester" water profile (Greater Manchester):
Ca^{2+}: 10 ppm, Mg^{2+}: 1 ppm, Na^+: 7 ppm, Cl^-: 6 ppm, SO_4^{2-}: 15 ppm, Alkalinity (as $CaCO_3$): 15 ppm, pH: 7.24

HOPS

0.5 oz. (14 g) Mt. Hood (6.5% AA) @ 60 min.

YEAST

1 sachet (10 g, or 0.3 oz.) Mangrove Jack's M15 Empire Ale yeast

BREWING NOTES

1. With 4.5 gal. (17 L) of strike water, first mash in the rice malts only at 190°F (88°C), adding the Termamyl SC DS. Rest at this temperature for 20 min., stirring once halfway through.
2. Mash in remaining grains and 0.5 gal. (1.89 L) of cold water to reach 125°F (52°C). Add the Ceremix Flex and Ondea Pro, along with brewing salts to match suggested water profile. Let rest for 20 min.
3. Raise mash temperature to 145°F (63°C) and rest for 45 min.
4. Raise mash temperature again to 175°F (79°C) and rest for 20 mins.
5. Recirculate wort over grain bed until clear wort is obtained. Sparge at 180°F (82°C).
6. Boil for 60 min. with Mt. Hood hops. Add a pinch of Irish moss and any desired gluten-free yeast nutrient with 15 min. left in the boil.
7. Chill to 68°F (20°C) and pitch yeast.
8. Ferment at 68°F (20°C) for two weeks. Once terminal gravity has been reached, cold crash for three days or until the beer is clear of suspended yeast.
9. Package and carbonate to 2.3 vol. CO_2.

BURTON'S BEAST ENGLISH IPA

Gluten-Free English-Style India Pale Ale

Contributed by Robert Keifer

Having only tried a few English-style IPAs before going gluten free, I have always been intrigued by this style due to the counterpoint it provides to American-style IPA. Whereas many of the American IPAs I have tried were either citrusy or dank resin bombs, English-style IPAs seemed to bring more of a rich maltiness, with an ability to be great when dry due to the more subtle and less in-your-face hop note that was still hop forward. For this recipe, I used some British hops like Target (for bittering) and Challenger (for character), but I also added some hops to the late boil and dry hop that are more commonly featured in New World pale ales and hazy IPAs—Galaxy, Belma, and El Dorado—the thought being to provide a lovely stone fruit aroma paired with a spicy, bitter fruit flavor note on the palette.

For 5 US gal. (18.9 L)

Original gravity: 1.062 (15.2°P)
Final gravity: 1.010 (2.6°P)
Color: 7–8 SRM (14–16 EBC)

IBU: 65
ABV: 6.8%

FERMENTABLES

5.0 lb. (2.27 kg) Eckert pale rice malt
6.0 lb. (2.72 kg) Grouse pale millet malt
1.0 lb. (0.45 kg) Grouse Munich millet malt 2.5°L

0.5 lb. (0.23 kg) Grouse caramel millet malt 4°L
4 oz. (113 g) Grouse roasted Cara Millet malt 15–40°L

ENZYMES

12.75 mL Ceremix® Flex (equivalent to 1 mL/lb. grain, or 2.2 mL/kg)
12.75 mL Ondea® Pro (1 mL/lb., or 2.2 mL/kg)

WATER

Aim for a "Burton-on-Trent" water profile:
Ca^{2+}: 287 ppm, Mg^{2+}: 41 ppm, Na^+: 113 ppm, K^+: 7 ppm, Cl^-: 85 ppm, SO_4^{2-}: 764 ppm, Alkalinity (as $CaCO_3$): 229 ppm

HOPS

1.0 oz. (28 g) Target (10% AA) @ 60 min.
1.0 oz. (28 g) Galaxy (11%–16% AA) @ whirlpool (20 min. @ 190°F, 88°C)
1.0 oz. (28 g) Challenger (6.5%–9% AA) @ whirlpool (20 min. @ 190°F, 88°C)
0.5 oz. (14 g) Galaxy (11%–16% AA) @ dry hop
0.5 oz. (14 g) Belma (10% AA) @ dry hop
0.5 oz. (14 g) El Dorado (14%–16% AA) @ dry hop

YEAST

3 sachets (33 g, or 1.16 oz.) Lallemand Nottingham ale yeast (rehydrated)

BREWING NOTES

1. Heat 5 gal. (18.9 L) of strike water to 135°F (57°C) and mash in with entire grist; mash temperature should be 125°F (52°C). Adjust pH to 5.2. Add Ceremix Flex and Ondea Pro and rest 25 min. at 125°F (52°C).
2. Raise mash temperature to 150°F (66°C) and rest 25 min. again.
3. Raise mash temperature to 175°F (79°C) and hold for an additional 25 min.
4. Mash out at 180°F (82°C) for 10 min., then perform sparge.

Continued >

5. Boil for 60 min. with Target hops. Add a pinch of Irish moss and any desired gluten-free yeast nutrient with 15 min. left in the boil.
6. At the end of the boil, chill wort down to 190°F (88°C), and whirlpool with Galaxy and Challenger hops.
7. Chill to 68°F (20°C) and pitch yeast.
8. Ferment at 68°F (20°C) for two weeks. Once active fermentation is finished, dry hop with Galaxy, Belma, and El Dorado.
9. Cold condition, keg, and serve. Carbonate to 2.4 vol. CO_2.

HELLO DARKNESS DRY OAT STOUT

Gluten-Free Dry Irish Stout

Contributed by Brian Newcomb (Gluten Free Brew Supply)

Brian Newcomb, owner of Gluten Free Brew Supply, says, "I love a good stout with a silky body. A huge dose of gluten-free malted oats combined with the sorghum malt base and specialty malts and highlighted with hops results in a classic DARK dry oat stout."

For 5 US gal. (18.9 L)

Original gravity: 1.045 (11.2°P)
Final gravity: 1.006 (1.5°P)
Color: 59 SRM (116 EBC)

IBU: 25
ABV: 5.1%

FERMENTABLES

5.0 lb. (2.27 kg) red sorghum malt
4.0 lb. (1.80 kg) gluten-free oat malt
1.5 lb. (0.68 kg) Eckert biscuit rice malt 5°L
1.5 lb. (0.68 kg) Grouse pale buckwheat malt

1.0 lb. (0.45 kg) Grouse chocolate roast millet malt
1.0 lb. (0.45 kg) Grouse medium roast millet malt
1.0 lb. (0.45 kg) Grouse Caramel 120L millet malt
0.5 lb. (0.23 kg) Eckert Pitch Black rice malt

ENZYMES

15.5 mL Ceremix® Flex (equivalent to 1 mL/lb. grain, or 2.2 mL/kg)
15.5 mL Ondea® Pro (1 mL/lb., or 2.2 mL/kg)

WATER

Aim for a "Kilkenny" water profile:
Ca^{2+}: 35 ppm, Mg^{2+}: 8 ppm, Na^+: 46 ppm, Cl^-: 77 ppm, SO_4^{2-}: 21 ppm, $CaCO_3$: 90 ppm, pH: 5.6

HOPS

0.5 oz. (14 g) Northern Brewer (9.5% AA) @ 60 min.
0.5 oz. (14 g) Northern Brewer (9.5% AA) @ 30 min.
0.5 oz. (14 g) Fuggle (4.5% AA) @ 30 min.
0.5 oz. (14 g) Fuggle (4.5% AA) @ 15 min.
1.0 oz. (28 g) cocoa nibs @ 15 min.

YEAST

1 sachet (11 g, or 0.39 oz.) Lallemand Nottingham ale yeast

BREWING NOTES

1. Heat strike water to 135°F (57°C) and mash in with entire grist; mash temperature should be 125°F (52°C). Add Ceremix Flex and Ondea Pro and rest for 25 min. at 125°F (52°C).
2. Raise mash to 150°F (66°C) and rest 25 min.
3. Raise mash to 175°F (79°C) and hold for an additional 25 min.
4. Mash out at 180°F (82°C) for 10 min., then perform sparge and boil.
5. Chill wort to 60°F (16°C), and pitch yeast.
6. Ferment at 60–65°F (16–18°C) for 7–10 days, then cold crash and package.

STURDY ALE WINE

Gluten-Free Ale (or "Barley-") Wine

Contributed by Jason Yerger of Mutantis Brewing, Portland, OR

Jason Yerger took up homebrewing in his late 20s, just a few years after he was diagnosed with celiac disease. As a dyed-in-the-wool Bay Area beer geek, he could not abide the lack of any craft gluten-free beer in the late 2000s and set out to brew it himself. As he got more and more serious about the science of gluten-free brewing, he began closing the gap between his brews and the gluten-containing beers he fondly remembered.

In 2013, after building a modest internet presence via his blog *Brewing Beyond Barley* (https://beyondbarley.com), Jason relocated to Seattle to become the head brewer at Ghostfish Brewing Company, Washington's first dedicated gluten-free brewery. While there, he won numerous awards and helped Ghostfish rapidly grow to be a national brand. Jason left in 2018 to launch a consulting company, followed by opening Mutantis Brewery & Bottle Shop (https://mutantis.beer) in Portland, OR, in November of 2020. All Mutantis recipes and processes are "open source," because Jason believes sharing knowledge is the best thing for the gluten-free brewing industry.

Jason explains his inspiration for Sturdy Ale Wine:

> This beer is meant to demonstrate that gluten-free beers can be every bit as rich and malt-forward as beers made from barley. Amber rice malt is somewhere between a true amber malt and a crystal malt, and packs in tons of sweet caramel flavors. Munich millet malt, on the other hand, is more of an English pale ale malt and gives a subtle strawberry-like note to the aroma. The Biscuit 15L (also known as "Medium Biscuit") gives a deep toasty note, and the Caramel 90L millet malt deepens the color and emphasizes the caramelly richness of the beer. A bit of brown sugar in the boil helps boost the gravity and lighten the body without detracting from the rich aroma. The hop quantities can also be adjusted to taste; it's a very rich beer and could stand up to a heavier hop schedule.

For 5 US gal. (18.9 L)

Original gravity: 1.098 (23.3°P)
Final gravity: 1.020 (5.1°P)
Color: 17 SRM (34 EBC)

IBU: 71
ABV: 10.5%

FERMENTABLES

9.0 lb. (4.08 kg) Grouse Munich millet malt
9.0 lb. (4.08 kg) Eckert amber rice malt
1.0 lb. (0.45 kg) Eckert biscuit rice malt 15°L

0.5 lb. (0.23 kg) Grouse Caramel 90L millet malt
0.5 lb. (0.23 kg) brown sugar (added at start of boil)

ENZYMES

15 mL Termamyl® SC (equivalent to 0.77 mL/lb. grain, or 1.7 mL/kg)
20 mL Ceremix® Flex (1.03 mL/lb. grain, or 2.3 mL/kg)
22 mL Ondea® Pro (1.1 mL/lb. grain, or 2.4 mL/kg)

WATER

Ca^{2+}: 54 ppm, Mg^{2+}: 17 ppm, Na^+ 17 ppm, SO_4^{2-} 118 ppm, Cl^- 54 ppm, HCO_3^- 48 ppm

HOPS

1.0 oz. (28 g) CTZ (14.0% AA) @ 90 min.
1.0 oz. (28 g) Cascade (5.5% AA) @ 15 min.
2.0 oz. (28 g) Chinook (13.0% AA) @ 0 min. (steep for 15 min.)

ADDITIONAL INGREDIENTS
1 tablet Whirlfloc @ 10 min.

YEAST
2 sachets (22 g, or 0.78 oz.) Lallemand Nottingham ale yeast

BREWING NOTES
1. Mash in so that mash temperature hits 125°F (52°C), then add all three enzymes. Raise mash temperature to 145°F (63°C) over 20 min., then hold for 45 min.
2. Raise mash temperature to 175°F (79°C) over 20 min., then hold for 30 min.
3. Sparge with 209°F (98°C) water. Collect 7 gal. (26.5 L) of pre-boil wort into the boil kettle.
4. Boil 90 minutes, adding CTZ hops at the start of the boil and Cascade with 15 min. left in the boil. Add Chinook hops at flameout and let sit for 15 min.
5. Chill wort to 65°F (18°C) and pitch yeast.
6. Ferment 14 days at 65°F (18°C).
7. Condition 5 days at 38°F (3°C).
8. Carbonate to 2.1 vol. CO_2.

MILLETWINE
Gluten-Free Ale Wine

Contributed by Robert Keifer

The first gluten-free version of an ale wine that I ever tried was Grandpa's Nap from Evasion brewing in McMinnville, OR. Head brewer Ben Acord makes amazing, big beers, and the medal-winning MilletWine is really something special (2019 GABF Bronze, Gluten-Free Beer category). To give it a specific style label like ale wine feels like caging a wild animal, as this beer is majestic, with a rich, deep caramel from kettle caramelization. Original versions of MilletWine involved only pale millet malt and boiling the first runnings down to half volume; this was repeated until the fermentor was full. The beer was barrel aged to impart lovely boozy, sweet vanilla, and roast notes and it had a pleasing stickiness to it.

For this recipe, I took that same inspiration of a longer boil, but I focused on being able to get to the target starting gravity all in one batch. I also added certain character malts that will accentuate certain flavors like raisin and caramel, which will work well with the English ale yeast used. Because the starting gravity is so high, you will need to make sure you pitch enough yeast to ferment all the way to terminal gravity. Some yeast stress is to be expected, which may necessitate aging the beer as these stresses can often manifest as fusel alcohols (i.e., hot and boozy). I have brewed a batch or two of this beer that definitely benefited from extra aging.

For 5.5 US gal. (20.8 L)

Original gravity: 1.100 (23.8°P)
Final gravity: 1.012 (3.1°P)
Color: 14–15 SRM (28–30 EBC)

IBU: 23
ABV: 11.5%

FERMENTABLES*

6.00 lb. (2.72 kg) Grouse pale millet malt
6.25 lb. (2.83 kg) Grouse Vienna millet malt
4.25 lb. (1.93 kg) Eckert pale rice malt

0.50 lb. (0.23 kg) Eckert James' Brown rice malt
0.50 lb. (0.23 kg) Eckert crystal rice malt
0.50 lb. (0.23 kg) Grouse Red Wing millet malt

ENZYMES

18 mL Ceremix® Flex (equivalent to 1 mL/lb. grain, or 2.2 mL/kg),
18 mL Termamyl® (1 mL/lb., or 2.2 mL/kg)
18 mL Ondea® Pro (1 mL/lb., or 2.2 mL/kg)

HOPS

2 oz. (57 g) East Kent Golding (5.5% AA) @ 60 min.

ADDITIONAL INGREDIENTS

1 tsp Irish moss @ 15 min.
0.08 oz. (2.26 g) Yeastex 61 yeast nutrient (allergen warning: contains soy) @ 15 min.†

YEAST

3 sachets (30 g, or 1.1 oz.) Mangrove Jack's M15 Empire Ale yeast

BREWING NOTES

1. Perform a rising-step mash. Mash in, add all three enzymes, and rest at 125°F (52°C) for 20 min. Raise mash temperature to 145°F (63°C) and rest for 45 min. Raise mash temperature to 175°F (79°C) and rest for 20 min.
2. Sparge, collecting about 7.5 gal. (28.4 L). Boil wort for 2 hours, aiming for a finishing volume of 5.5 gal. (20.8 L) or less. Boiling for longer will develop richer notes, but you will want to add the hops at 60 min. regardless of boil length to avoid overbittering the beer.

3. Chill wort to 68°F (20°C), and pitch yeast.
4. Ferment at 68°F (20°C) for 21 days.
5. Cold crash over 3 days, then package. Bottle conditioning is ideal but kegging and force carbonating works as well. Carbonate to 2.4 vol. CO_2.

ADDITIONAL NOTES

* Adding sugar and syrups during the boil is a great idea if you do not extract all the necessary sugars from the grains.
† You can add up to 1 whole teaspoon of Yeastex depending on what mash method or ingredients you use; for example, doing a partial mash with sorghum syrup.

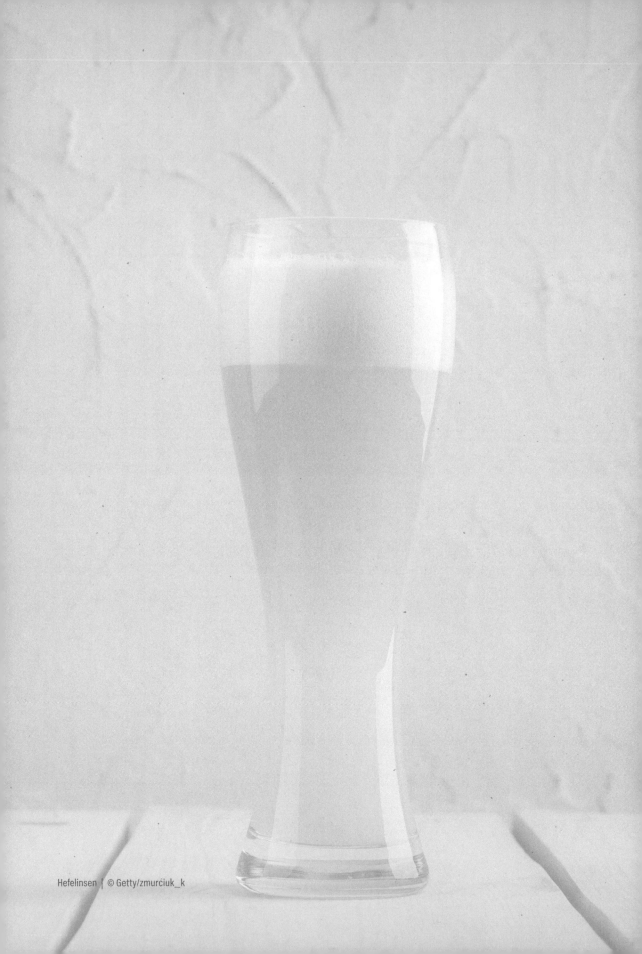

7

Continental European Styles

Continental European styles, whether lager or ale, have such a rich culture built around them that they have become the very bedrock of what most people think of when they think of beer, or should I say *Bier* (or *pivo*)? In some European towns, the very fabric of daily life involves beer. Sure, the crafty IPAs and other styles that have become popular nowadays have their place in beer culture, but these European styles are timeless. Characterized by malt-forward flavors and aromas accentuated with noble hops, with a balanced taste profile and essential drinkability at the center of it all, these beers are near and dear to many a beer lover's heart.

Even if something as strict as the age-old *Reinheitsgebot* couldn't possibly apply here, many of the following recipes still adhere to a simple format of water, malt, hops, and, of course, yeast. Where I had the information on brewing water, I have included it, although that was not always possible.

You will notice, however, that some recipes do feature unmalted ingredients such as lentils, dextrose, or white sorghum syrup. As we have spoken about, adding unmalted or non-grain ingredients is sometimes the best strategy for achieving true-to-style flavors and textures; in the case of additional sugar adjuncts, this is to achieve the correct starting gravity. If you are setting out to make all-grain high-gravity brews of one or two of these recipes, I suggest double-batching, with several first runnings from multiple mashes being run into the boil kettle to achieve the starting gravity you are aiming for.

HEFELINSEN
Gluten-Free Hefeweisen

Contributed by Robert Keifer

I tried my first Hefelinsen when I met Ed Golden at the 2018 Homebrew Con™ in Portland, OR. (That was also the first year that I did a seminar on gluten-free brewing.) When I tried the Hefelinsen, I realized how truly little I knew about gluten-free brewing. There was so much more to learn about gluten-free brewing than I had originally thought, and that inspired me to do the research for this book.

Ed uses a rising decantation mash (p. 89) for his original recipe, as well as homemade malt, and I would recommend taking those steps as well if you feel you are experienced enough. For this recipe, I have included ingredients that can be sourced from US maltsters Grouse and Eckert (and the grocery store for the lentils), and used a rising-step mash regime that relies on exogenous enzymes, assuming the average homebrewer has the ability to do a rising-step mash. Refer to chapter 5 for the proper steps to take when using the decantation method, a single infusion mash, or falling temperature step mash.

For 5.5 gallons (20.8 L)

Original gravity: 1.045 (11.2°P)
Final gravity: 1.010 (2.6°P)
Color: 2 SRM (4 EBC)

IBU: 12
ABV: 4.5%

FERMENTABLES
4.0 lb. (1.8 kg) Grouse pale millet malt
1.0 lb. (0.45 kg) Grouse Vienna millet malt
4.0 lb. (1.8 kg) Eckert biscuit rice malt
0.5 lb. (0.23 kg) lentils (any color will do)

ENZYMES
11 mL Ceremix® Flex (equivalent to 1.2 mL/lb. grain, or 2.6 mL/kg)
11 mL Termamyl® (1.2 mL/lb. grain, or 2.6 mL/kg)
11 mL Ondea® Pro (1.2 mL/lb. grain, or 2.6 mL/kg)

HOPS
1 oz. (28 g) Hallertauer Mittelfrüher (4% AA) @ 60 min.

ADDITIONAL INGREDIENTS
small pinch Irish moss @ 15 min.
0.08 oz. (2.3 g) Yeastex 61 yeast nutrient (allergen warning: contains soy) @ 15 min.

YEAST
1 sachet (11.5 g, or 0.4 oz.) Fermentis SafAle™ WB-06

BREWING NOTES
1. Perform a rising-step mash. Mash in using 4 gal. (15.1 L) strike water, add all three enzymes, and rest at 125°F (52°C) for 20 min. Mash pH should come in at 5.2–5.3.
2. Raise mash temperature to 145°F (63°C) and rest for 45 min. Raise mash temperature to 175°F (79°C) and rest for 20 min.
3. Before the mash is finished, preheat sparge water to 180°F (82°C). At the end of the mash, perform your sparge to collect a pre-boil volume of approximately 6 gal. (22.7 L).
4. When the boil is complete, cool the wort and transfer to the fermentor. Pitch yeast and ferment at 74°F (18°C) until specific gravity is stable and fermentation is complete (approximately 14 days, or until active fermentation is over).
5. Cold crash and package. Or, for more traditional results, package with live yeast. Carbonate to 2.6 vol CO_2.

TO HELLES AND BACK
Gluten-Free German Helles Exportbier
Contributed by Bierly Brewing, McMinnville, OR

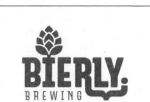

Bierly Brewing began brewing commercially in 2016 as Oregon's second gluten-free brewery, but the owners' gluten-free roots go back much further. Husband-and-wife team JP and Amelia both live gluten free, JP being diagnosed with celiac disease in 2010 and Amelia having lived with celiac disease her whole life. As a homebrewer, JP was using gluten-free ingredients as early as 2006, before an internship in 2012 with Heater Allen Brewing in McMinnville, OR led him eventually to running a small family brewery of his own with Amelia.

First located in a dedicated gluten-free restaurant in Philomath, OR, in 2018 Bierly Brewing moved to their own facility in McMinnville, opening a tasting room serving Amelia's innovative gluten-free baked and fried foods, as much of a draw to the tasting room as the beer. In 2021, Bierly completed renovations on a building in McMinnville's Historic Downtown and moved the brewery and tasting room into the new, larger space.

Still head brewer at Bierly, JP is recognized by his colleagues as a top-notch brewer and mentor to professional brewers and homebrewers alike. His recipe here demonstrates how a classic, delicious style of beer can be brewed gluten free without a complicated grain bill.

For 5.5 gallons (20.8 L)

Original gravity: 1.057 (14°P)
Final gravity: 1.012 (3.1°P)
Color: 8 SRM (16 EBC)

IBU: 23
ABV: 5.9%

FERMENTABLES
6.25 lb. (2.83 kg) Grouse Vienna millet malt
4.25 lb. (1.93 kg) Eckert pale rice malt

ENZYMES
11 mL Ceremix® Flex (equivalent to 1.05 mL/lb. grain, or 2.3 mL/kg)
11 mL Termamyl® (1.05 mL/lb. grain, or 2.3 mL/kg)
11 mL Ondea® Pro (1.05 mL/lb. grain, or 2.3 mL/kg)

WATER
Based on McMinnville, OR water profile:
Ca^{2+}: 8.65 ppm, Mg^{2+}: 2.30 ppm, Na^+: 8.32 ppm, Cl^-: 6.2 ppm, SO_4^{2-}: 8.70 ppm, Alkalinity (as $CaCO_3$): 19 ppm, pH: 7.28

HOPS
2 oz. (57 g) Tettnang (3.1% AA) @ first wort hop

ADDITIONAL INGREDIENTS
small pinch Irish moss @ 15 min.
0.08 oz. (2.3 g) Yeastex 61 yeast nutrient (allergen warning: contains soy) @ 15 min.

YEAST
1 sachet (11.5 g, or 0.4 oz.) Fermentis SafLager™ W-34/70

Continued >

BREWING NOTES

1. Perform a rising-step mash. Mash in using 4 gal. (15.1 L) strike water, add all three enzymes, and rest at 125°F (52°C) for 20 min. Mash pH should come in at 5.2–5.3.
2. Raise mash temperature to 145°F (63°C) and rest for 45 min. Raise mash temperature to 175°F (79°C) and rest for 20 min.
3. Before the mash is finished, preheat sparge water to 180°F (82°C). At the end of the mash, perform your sparge to collect a pre-boil volume of approximately 6 gal. (22.7 L).
4. When the boil is complete, cool the wort to 68°F (20°C) and transfer to the fermentor. Pitch yeast and ferment at 68°F (20°C) for 14 days.
5. Cold age the beer for 30–45 days, or until the liquid is clear. Carbonate to 2.5 vol. CO_2.

CIRCUIT BREAKER MILLET LAGER
Gluten-Free Lager

Contributed by Suspect Brewing from Scotland

This is the flagship beer from Suspect Brewing and it is brewed for mass appeal in the gluten-free category in the UK. At this time, it is one of only two UK-based breweries using 100% gluten-free ingredients, the other being the UK-based maltster The AltGrain Co.

Suspect Brewing uses a rising step mash for this recipe, but you could employ a falling step mash (see chapter 5 for guidance based on which malts you are using).

For 5.5 US gal. (20.8 L)

Original gravity (est.): 1.042 (10.5°P)
Final gravity (est.): 1.008–1.010 (2.1–2.6°P)
Color: 3 SRM (6 EBC)

IBU: 29
ABV (est.): 4.2%–4.4%

FERMENTABLES

6.6 lb. (3.0 kg) pale millet malt
14 oz. (0.4 kg) pale buckwheat malt
7 oz. (0.2 kg) Munich millet malt

7 oz. (0.2 kg) dextrose
7 oz. (0.2 kg) rice hulls (to aid in wort separation)

ENZYMES

11 mL Ceremix® Flex (equivalent to 1.4 mL/lb. grain, or 3.1 mL/kg)
11 mL Termamyl® (1.4 mL/lb. grain, or 3.1 mL/kg)
11 mL Ondea® Pro (1.4 mL/lb. grain, or 3.1 mL/kg)

WATER

Pilsen-type soft water profile—very little salts at all

HOPS

0.45 oz. (13 g) Magnum (11.1% AA) @ 60 min.
1.8 oz. (53 g) Saaz (3.5% AA) @ 10 min.

YEAST

1 sachet (11.5 g, or 0.4 oz.) Fermentis SafAle™ K-97

BREWING NOTES

1. Perform a rising-step mash. Mash in using 4 gal. (15.1 L) strike water, add all three enzymes, and rest at 125°F (52°C) for 20 min. Mash pH should come in at 5.2–5.3.
2. Raise mash temperature to 145°F (63°C) and rest for 45 min. Raise mash temperature to 175°F (79°C) and rest for 20 min.
3. Before the mash is finished, preheat sparge water to 180°F (82°C). At the end of the mash, perform your sparge to collect a pre-boil volume of approximately 6 gal. (22.7 L).
4. When the boil is complete, cool the wort to 59°F (15°C) and transfer to the fermentor. Pitch yeast and ferment at 59°F (15°C) for one week.
5. Lager the fermenting beer at 43°F (6°C) for two weeks.
6. Carbonate to 2.6 vol CO_2.

BAKER'S KÖLSCH

Gluten-Free Kölsch

Contributed by Ben Fowler

Kölsch has long been a favorite style of Ben Fowler. While Kölsch is an ale, it shares many of the refreshing and easy-drinking characteristics of a lager. This recipe is pretty balanced and lets the Kölsch yeast's unique flavors shine. You will always find this on tap at Ben's house!

Batch Size: 5.5 gal (20.8 L)

Original gravity: 1.043 (10.7°P)   **IBU:** 25
Final gravity: 1.008 (2.1°P)   **ABV:** 4.6%
Color: 4 SRM (8 EBC)

FERMENTABLES

7.5 lb. (3.4 kg) Grouse pale millet
2.0 lb. (0.91 kg) Eckert biscuit rice malt
0.5 lb. (0.23 kg) Grouse pale buckwheat malt

4.0 oz. (113 g) Grouse caramel millet malt
4.0 oz. (113 g) Grouse Cara Millet

ENZYMES

15 mL Termamyl® (equivalent to 1.4 mL/lb. grain, or 3.2 mL/kg)
15 mL SEBAmyl® L (1.4 mL/lb. grain, or 3.2 mL/kg)
11 mL Ondea® Pro (1.1 mL/lb. grain, or 2.3 mL/kg)

HOPS

1.5 oz. (43 g) Saaz (3% AA) @ 60 min.
1.0 oz. (28 g) Hallertauer (4% AA) @ 15 min.

ADDITIONAL INGREDIENTS

4 tsp yeast nutrient @ 15 min.
1 Whirfloc tablet @ 15 min.

YEAST

Propagate Lab MIP-510 Kölsch yeast, or 1 sachet either Fermentis SafAle™ K-97 (11.5 g, or 0.4 oz.)
   or Lallemand LalBrew Köln™ (11 g, or 0.39 oz.)

BREWING NOTES

1. Add 13.2 qts (3.28 gal.) strike water (1.25 qt/lb), add the Termamyl, and mash at 185°F (85°C) for 60 min.
2. Add 2–3 qt. (1.9–2.8 L) cold water to the mash until the temperature drops to 145°F (63°C). Add SEBAmyl L and Ondea Pro and rest for 90 min. Mash pH should come in at 5.2–5.3.
3. Before the mash is finished, preheat sparge water to 180°F (82°C). At the end of the mash, perform your sparge to collect a pre-boil volume of approximately 6 gal. (22.7 L).
4. When the boil is complete, cool the wort to 70°F (21.1°C) and transfer to the fermentor. Pitch yeast and ferment at 67°F (19°C) for 6 days.
5. Rack to secondary and cold crash. Keg and serve. Carbonate to 2.5 vol CO_2.

HENRY'S VIENNA LAGER
Gluten-Free Vienna Lager

Contributed by Cale Baldwin

One of the beer styles Cale missed most when moving to gluten-free brewing was a nice crisp lager. Cale's hope was to create a recipe that provided a drinkable lager using light noble hops. He named this brew after his eight-year-old son Henry, who's always the assistant brewer in the garage. This is the anti-IPA, with low hopping and rich creamy mouthfeel. If you've been missing lagers, give this recipe a try and you'll not be disappointed.

For 6 US gal. (22.7 L)

Original gravity: 1.058 (14.3°P)
Final gravity: 1.010 (2.6°P)
Color: 8 SRM (17 EBC)

IBU: 32
ABV: 6.29%

FERMENTABLES

4.0 lb. (1.8 kg) Grouse pale millet malt
4.0 lb. (1.8 kg) Grouse Vienna millet malt
1.0 lb. (0.45 kg) Grouse Munich millet malt
1.0 lb. (0.45 kg) Grouse Goldfinch Millet Malt
2.0 lb. (0.91 kg) Eckert biscuit rice malt

2.0 lb. (0.91 kg) Grouse pale buckwheat malt
0.5 lb. (0.23 kg) Grouse Cara Millet malt
1.0 lb. (0.45 kg) rice hulls (to aid in wort
   separation)

ENZYMES

16 mL Ceremix® Flex (equivalent to 1.1 mL/lb. grain, or 2.4 mL/kg)
16 mL Ondea® Pro (1.1 mL/lb. grain, or 2.4 mL/kg)

HOPS

2 oz. (57 g) Hallertau Hersbrucker (3.5% AA) @ 60 min.
1 oz. (28 g) Hallertau Hersbrucker (3.5% AA) @ 15 min.

ADDITIONAL INGREDIENTS

2 tbsp (30 g) yeast nutrient @ 15 min.
1 Whirfloc® tablet @ 15 min.
2 tsp calcium chloride (if RO water)

YEAST

1 sachet (11.5 g, or 0.4 oz.) Fermentis SafLager™ S-23

BREWING NOTES

1. Mash in using 6 gal. (22.7 L) 155°F (68°C) strike water, add Ceremix Flex and Ondea Pro and rest at 145°F (63°C) for 60 min.
2. SLOWLY raise mash to 175°F (79°C) and rest for 30 min.
3. Sparge with 12 qt. (11.4 L) of 180°F (82°C) water. Collect 6 gal. (22.7 L) into the boil kettle.
4. Boil for one hour, adding hops per schedule, then cool the wort to 60°F (15.5°C).
5. Pitch yeast and ferment at 54°F (12°C) until fermentation is nearly complete.
6. Perform diacetyl rest by ramping up to 60-65°F (16-18°C) for two weeks.
7. Lager at 35°F (2°C) for 30 days.
8. Keg and serve. Carbonate to 2.3 vol. CO_2.

DARKNESS TAKES FLIGHT
Gluten-Free Dark Czech Lager

Contributed by Brian Newcomb

Brian Newcomb was challenged to make a dark lager by his friend and Bierly Brewing head brewer, JP (p. 111).

For 5.5 US gal. (20.8 L)

Original gravity: 1.055 (13.8°P)
Final gravity: 1.006 (1.5°P)
Color: 18 SRM

IBU: 36
ABV: 6.43%

FERMENTABLES
1.0 lb. (0.45 kg) Grouse Red Wing millet malt
1.0 lb. (0.45 kg) yellow corn malt
2.0 lb. (0.91 kg) Eckert biscuit rice 4.8°L
2.0 lb. (0.91 kg) Grouse Caramel 90L millet malt
6.0 lb. (2.72 kg) red sorghum malt (available from Gluten Free Brew Supply)

ENZYMES
16 mL Ceremix® Flex (equivalent to 2.7 mL/lb. grain, or 5.9 mL/kg)
16 mL Ondea® Pro (2.7 mL/lb. grain, or 5.9 mL/kg)

WATER
Aim for a Pilsen-style profile:
Ca^{2+}: 7 ppm, Mg^{2+}: 3 ppm, Na^+: 2 ppm, Cl^-: 5 ppm, SO_4^{2-}: 5 ppm, HCO_3^-: 25 ppm

HOPS
0.5 oz. (7 g) Loral (11.5% AA) @ 60 min.
0.5 oz. (21 g) Loral (11.5% AA) @ 10 min.

YEAST
2 sachets (23 g, 0.8 oz.) Fermentis SafLager™ W-34/70

BREWING NOTES
1. Mash in at 125°F (52°C) with 24 qt. (22.7 L) of water. Add both the Ceremix Flex and Ondea Pro when temperature reaches 145°F (63°C) and rest for 60 min.
2. Raise mash to 175°F (79°C) and rest for 30 min. Sparge with 12 qt. (11.4 L) water heated to 180°F (82°C) until you obtain 6 gal. pre-boiled wort.
3. When mashing is complete, collect the first third of the mash runnings into a separate bucket and set aside. Add the other two thirds to the kettle and heat in preparation for the boil.
4. Boil for 60 min., adding hops per schedule, then cool wort to 60°F (15.5°C).
5. Pitch yeast and ferment at 60–65°F (16–18°C) for 2 weeks.
6. Cold condition at 35°F (2°C) for 4 weeks. Carbonate to 2.3 vol. CO_2 before serving.

DEVIL'S IN THE DOPPELBOCK

Gluten-Free Doppelbock *Contributed by Reid Ackerman and Brian Thiel, Ghostfish Brewing, Seattle, WA*

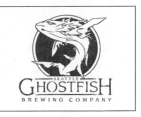

This recipe is for a homebrew version of 5th Anniversary Doppelbock from Ghostfish. What better way to celebrate an anniversary than with a gorgeous and luxurious German doppelbock! 5th Anniversary Doppelbock is a malt-forward German-style lager, exhibiting notes of caramelized pear, noble hop spice, and a malty aroma. The rich malt and full mouthfeel also showcase notes of maple, raisin, toffee, and light cognac/brandy.

I wasn't fully aware of this beer's provenance when Ghostfish sent me their recipe for inclusion in this book. I messaged Reid saying, "I've tentatively named this beer 'Devil's in the Doppelbock' since you didn't send me all the relevant details for this beer, like its name..." To which Reid replied, "Let's keep that name, I love it!"

For 5 US gal. (18.9 L)

Original gravity: 1.074 (18°P) **IBU:** 20
Final gravity: 1.018 (4.5°P) **ABV:** 7.35%
Color: 16 SRM (32 EBC)

FERMENTABLES

1.25 lb. (0.57 kg) Briess white sorghum syrup
1.25 lb. (0.57 kg) rice extract syrup
1.25 lb. (0.57 kg) Grouse roasted Cara Millet malt
1.75 lb. (0.79 kg) Eckert amber rice malt
6.66 lb. (3.02 kg) Grouse Munich millet malt

ENZYMES

10 mL Ceremix® Flex (equivalent to 0.8 mL/lb. grain, or 1.8 mL/kg)
10 mL Ondea® Pro (0.8 mL/lb. grain, or 1.8 mL/kg)

HOPS

0.25 oz. (7 g) Hallertau Magnum (14.0% AA) @ 120 min.
0.5 oz. (14 g) Tettnanger (4.5% AA) @ 20 min.
0.5 oz. (14 g) Saaz (3.75% AA) @ 0 min., whirlpool 40 min.

ADDITIONAL INGREDIENTS

1 tablet Whirlfloc @ 10 min.

YEAST

3 packets (34.5 g, or 1.22 oz.) Fermentis SafLager™ W-34/70

BREWING NOTES

1. Strike at 145°F (63°C). Add Ceremix Flex and Ondea Pro. Rest for 60 min.
2. Raise to 175°F (79°C) and rest for 30 min.
3. Sparge with 12 qt. (11.4 L) of 180°F (82°C) water. Collect 7 gal. (26.5 L) into the boil kettle.
4. Boil for 120 min., adding hops per schedule, then cool the wort to 48°F (9°C).
5. Pitch the yeast and ferment at 48°F (9°C) until fermentation is nearly complete.
6. Perform diacetyl rest, ramping up to 65°F (18°C) for a couple of days.
7. Lager at 34°F (1°C) for 30 days.
8. Keg and serve. Carbonate to 2.5 vol. CO_2.

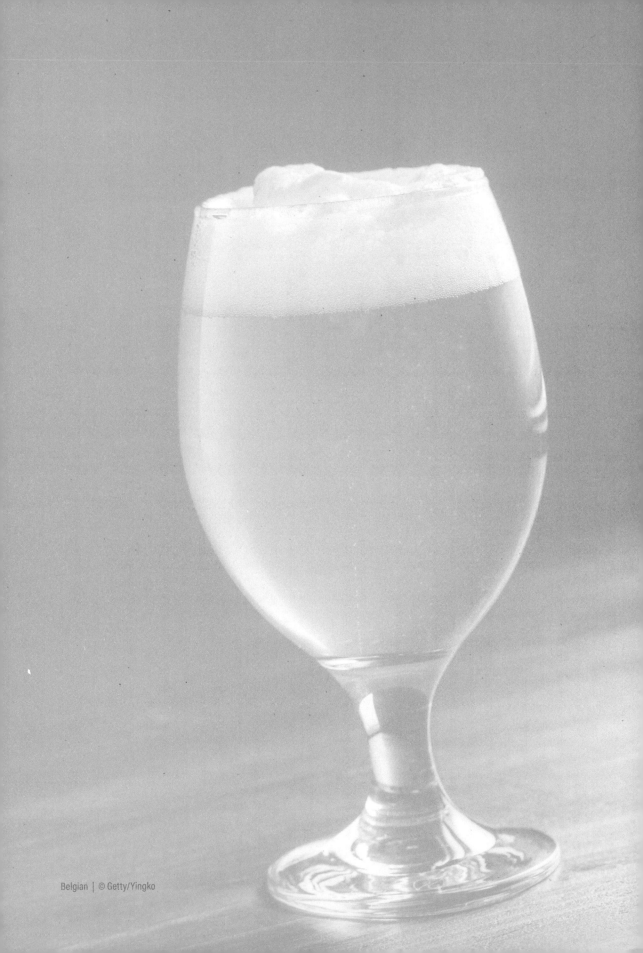

8

Belgian and French Styles

I love the way French and Belgian beers broaden the spectrum of what beer is. With a blending of traditional techniques and ingenuity (and even some wine-making techniques at times), you can achieve almost any flavor profile within these styles in gluten-free brewing. Where I had the information on brewing water, I have included it, although that was not always possible.

There are recipes incorporating many different base ingredients, from malted gluten-free grains to fruit to root vegetables, along with herbs and spices. Some are more playful than others and some are style-bending altogether. The key is these recipes use what's necessary to produce great beer, just like the brewers in Belgium and the north of France were doing.

MANGO WIT

Gluten-Free Fruited Belgian Witbier   *Contributed by Robert Keifer*

I've brewed this base beer recipe so many times. One of the first craft beers I ever tasted in my younger days was Hoegaarden; I then tried as many Belgian witbiers as I could until I went gluten free. It's one of my favorite styles. My wife loves anything fruity, so adding fruit to the fermentation every now and then made sense for me at home, and so, I fell in love with fruited witbier too. This kind of beer takes me to a place that a smoothie or mixed drink never could, and typically it is low enough in alcohol that I can drink it all day. I never seem to be able to brew enough witbier at home.

For 5.5 US gal. (20.8 L)

Original gravity: 1.050 (12.4°P)   **IBU:** 12
Final gravity: 1.010 (2.6°P)   **ABV:** 5.3% (up to 7.2% with fruit addition)
Color: 4–5 SRM

FERMENTABLES

6.0 lb. (2.72 kg) Grouse pale millet malt
2.0 lb. (0.91 kg) Eckert pale rice malt
1.5 lb. (0.68 kg) Grouse pale buckwheat
0.5 lb. (0.23 kg) Grouse Cara Millet malt

0.5 lb. (0.23 kg) Bob's Red Mill® Gluten Free Old Fashioned Rolled Oats (certified gluten free)
4.4 lb. (2.00 kg) mango puree

ENZYMES

10 mL Ondea® Pro enzyme (approx. 1.1 mL/lb.)
13 ml Ceremix® Flex (approx. 1.25 mL/lb.)

WATER

Ca^{2+}: 66 ppm, Mg^{2+}: 26 ppm, Na^+: 96 ppm, Cl^-: 94 ppm, SO_4^{2-}: 216 ppm HCO_3^-: 209 ppm

HOPS AND SPICES

1.00 oz. (28 g) US Tettnanger (3% AA) @ 45 min.
0.07 oz. (2 g) grains of paradise seeds, cracked or ground @ 15 min.
0.25 oz. (7 g) coriander, cracked or ground @ 15 min.
0.25 oz. (7 g) cardamom, ground @ 15 min. (optional)
0.25 oz. (7 g) juniper berries, whole @ 15 min. (optional)

YEAST

1 sachet (11.5 g, or 0.4 oz.) Fermentis SafAle™ WB-06

BREWING NOTES

1. Perform a rising-step mash. Heat 4.5 gal. (17 L) strike water. Mash in and rest at 125°F (52°C) for 15 min.
2. Raise mash temperature to 145°F (63°C) and rest for 30 min. Raise mash temperature to 175°F (79°C) and rest for 30 min. Raise mash temperature to 180°F (82°C) and rest for 15 min.
3. Before the mash is finished, preheat 1.5 gal. (5.7 L) sparge water to 180°F (82°C). At the end of the mash, perform your sparge to collect a pre-boil volume of approximately 6.5 gal. (24.6 L).
4. Boil for 60 min., adding hops and spices per schedule. When the boil is complete, cool the wort and transfer to the fermentor.
5. Pitch yeast and ferment at 85°F (29°C). At day 7, add fruit puree. Let sit for another 7–14 days.
6. Cold crash and package, although you can transfer with live yeast for a more traditional experience.

TRIPEL, YOUR PLEASURE
Gluten-Free Belgian Tripel

Contributed by Andrew Lavery, Geelong, VIC, Australia

After being diagnosed with celiac disease in 2003, Andrew Lavery adjusted to a gluten-free diet quite well, apart from the lack of beer. Cider just didn't cut it as a replacement, so Andrew dove headfirst into malting and brewing with gluten-free grains, drawing on a lot of research that had been done on sorghum and millet in Africa.

Andrew's experimentation and success at competitions convinced him to open O'Brien Brewing in 2004. O'Brien's Brown Ale earned a silver at the 2010 World Beer Cup® in the Gluten-Free Category and he also won several gold medals at the Australian International Beer Awards with beers he evolved from homebrew recipes. In 2017, Andrew moved into the world of traditional craft brewing, working at the Little Creatures/White Rabbit brewery in Geelong, where he delves into open fermentation, barrel sours, kettle sours, and IPAs. He continues to malt and brew gluten-free beers at home.

The inspiration for this tripel comes from the world of Belgian abbey beers that Andrew enjoyed prior to his diagnosis. Gold in color, with a white fluffy head, the aroma and flavor is balanced with spice, fruit, malt, and alcohol warmth. The Rakau hops add notes of stone fruit. For the mash, Andrew employs a modified decoction method called decantation, which I discuss in chapter 5. Briefly, it involves an initial mash step designed to pull out the grains' endogenous enzymes, preserving them for use later in the mash following a hotter gelatinization step. Pay careful attention to the brewing notes below.

For 5.2 US gal. (20 L)

Original gravity: 1.083 (20.0°P)
Final gravity: 1.010 (2.6°P)
Color: 6 SRM (12 EBC)

IBU: 33
ABV: 9.5%

FERMENTABLES
3.3 lb. (1.5 kg) pale maize malt*
8.8 lb. (4.0 kg) pale millet malt*

1.1 lb. (0.5 kg) Munich millet malt*
2.2 lb. (1.0 kg) dextrose (in the boil)

* Home made malts are used here. Commercial malts may not have sufficient β-amylase to attenuate. Gluten Free Home Brewing (https://www.glutenfreehomebrewing.com) has several tutorials in its resources section aimed at both the beginner and more advanced home-maltster.

ENZYMES
Decantation method—*see* Brewing Notes below and also p. 89

WATER
Ca²⁺: 150 ppm Mg²⁺: 1.9 ppm Na⁺: 7.7 ppm, Cl⁻: 150 ppm, SO₄²⁻: 75 ppm HCO₃⁻: 13 ppm

HOPS
0.7 oz. (20 g) Rakau (11.5% AA) @ 60 min.
0.7 oz. (20 g) Rakau (11.5% AA) @ whirlpool

YEAST
1 sachet (11.5 g, or 0.4 oz.) Fermentis SafAle™ BE-256

BREWING NOTES
1. Heat 3.96 gal. (15 L) water to 131°F (55°C) and mix in crushed malt and any brewing salts. Target mash pH between 5.2 and 5.5.
2. Conduct a protein rest at 126°F (52°C) for 15 min., allowing the grist to settle out.
3. Decant off 1.32 gal. (5.0 L) of clear liquid from the top of the mash. Place the decanted liquid in the fridge.

Continued >

4. Infuse the remaining mash with 1.32 gal. (5.0 L) of boiling water.
5. Heat mash to 158°F (70°C) and hold for 15 min. for partial conversion.
6. Heat mash to 194°F (90°C) and hold for 30 min. to gelatinize starch.
7. Cool mash to 158°F (70°C).
8. Add the refrigerated decanted liquid to the mash to achieve a mash temperature of 149°F (65°C). Hold mash at 149°F (65°C) for 60 min.
9. Heat mash to 167°F (75°C) and hold for 5 min., then sparge until 6.3 gal. (23.8 L) has been collected in the kettle.
10. Boil collected wort with hops as per schedule. After boil and whirlpool are finished, cool wort to 64.4°F (18°C).
11. Pitch yeast into 64.4°F (18°C) wort. Allow beer to free rise during fermentation; depending on ambient temperatures, it could get up to 80.6°F (27°C), which will cause the yeast to produce wonderful flavors and aromas.
12. Let ferment for up to 30 days. When done, cold condition for 3 days, package, and serve. For best results, bottle condition this beer and carbonate to 2.7–2.9 vol. CO_2. **Take care:** check the manufacturer's specification to ensure that your bottles can withstand higher levels of carbonation and avoid exploding bottles. Err on the side of caution since some standard beer bottles are not rated for high levels of carbonation and may explode.

BIERE DE GARDE
Gluten-Free Bière de Garde

Contributed by Robert Keifer

When I first started homebrewing, I fermented in PET plastic carboys. In 2018, for my Homebrew Con™ seminar, I wanted to bring a saison as an example beer for viewers of the presentation to taste. Wyeast graciously sent me a sample of 3711 French Saison that was not in the regular starter wort used in its commercial packets. It worked like a charm, and I was off brewing gluten-free saisons. Well, I didn't label the carboy until much too late and, as a result, 3711 made its way into all of my active PET carboys, as seemingly anything I brewed seemed to have saison characteristics. I decommissioned those carboys, but when we moved to a larger house, I decided to take these carboys out of storage and test what was in them with a spontaneous fermentation in each.

I filled each carboy with cooled wort and covered the opening with foil and a rubber band so no outside bugs or mites could get in but there was still some oxygen exposure. Within a week I noticed active fermentation; within another couple of weeks I even noticed pellicles forming. The aroma had notes of stone fruit and spicy esters. I enjoyed the resulting beers from this program so much that I further dedicated additional equipment to this spontaneous program at my house. In fact, the same culture is what we used when we scaled this recipe to our first bottle release at Divine Science Brewing, what we call Biere Du Divin. Lovely rich malt notes, with some acidity reminiscent of sourdough bread, some spicy esters, and an interesting sauvignon blanc note from the yeast interacting with the red sorghum malt—simply divine!

For 5.5 gallons (20.8 L)

Original gravity: 1.054 (13.3°P)
Final gravity: 1.006 (1.5°P)
Color: 6 SRM (12 EBC)

IBU: 18
ABV: 6.3%

FERMENTABLES
8.0 lb. (3.63 kg) red sorghum malt (avail. from Gluten Free Brew Supply)
1.0 lb. (0.45 kg) Eckert crystal rice malt
1.0 lb. (0.45 kg) Grouse Goldfinch Millet malt
1.0 lb. (0.45 kg) Grouse unmalted millet
0.5 lb. (0.23 kg) Grouse Caramel 90L millet malt
0.5 lb. (0.23 kg) Grouse Dutch Roast millet malt

ENZYMES
13 mL Ondea® Pro enzyme (approx. 1.1 mL/lb.)
15 mL Ceremix® Flex (approx. 1.25 mL/lb.)

WATER
Ca^{2+}: 66 ppm, Mg^{2+}: 26 ppm, Na^+: 96 ppm Cl^-: 94 ppm, SO_4^{2-}: 216 ppm, HCO_3^-: 209 ppm

HOPS
1 oz. (28 g) Tettnanger (3% AA) @ 60 min.

ADDITIONAL INGREDIENTS
small pinch Irish moss @ 15 min.
0.08 oz. (2.3 g) Yeastex 61 yeast nutrient (allergen warning: contains soy) @ 15 min.

YEAST
Option 1: 1 sachet (11.5 g, or 0.4 oz.) Fermentis SafAle™ T-58
Option 2: If you are comfortable spontaneously fermenting then go for it. Your results will likely vary from mine unless you know you have a *diastaticus* variant present.

Continued >

BREWING NOTES

1. Heat 4.5 gal. (17 L) strike water to 135°F (57°C; a liquor to grist ratio of 1.5 qt./lb.) mash in grains to achieve a rest temperature of 125°F (52°C), add enzymes and rest for 15 min.
2. Heat mash to 145°F (63°C), and perform second rest at 145°F (63°C) for 30 min.
3. Raise temperature to 175°F (79°C) and perform third rest at 175°F (79°C) for 30 min.
4. Raise temperature to 180°F (82°C) and begin vorlauf. Hold temperature at 180°F (82°C) for 15 min.
5. Sparge using 180°F (82°C) water. Sparge until 6.5 gal. (24.6 L) of wort are collected in the boil kettle.
6. Boil for 60 minutes with hops. Add a pinch of Irish moss and Yeastex 61 yeast nutrient with 15 min. left in the boil. After boil is done, chill wort to 68°F (20°C) and transfer to fermentor.
7. Pitch yeast and ferment at 68°F (20°C) for two weeks. Once terminal gravity has been reached, cold crash for three days or until the beer is clear of suspended yeast.
8. Package and carbonate to 2.9 vol. CO_2. **Take care:** check the manufacturer's specification to ensure that your bottles can withstand higher levels of carbonation and avoid exploding bottles. Err on the side of caution since some standard beer bottles are not rated for high levels of carbonation and may explode.

BRETT SAISON
Gluten-Free Saison with Secondary Fermentation

Contributed by Stuart Cole

Some styles of beer are hard to find in the commercial gluten-free beer world. That's true for saisons in general and "funky" (*Brettanomyces* or "Brett") versions in particular. Stuart Cole found that Propagate Lab in Colorado was producing a few runs of farmhouse/saison strains and a limited number of *Brettanomyces* strains on gluten-free media. Having access to these strains inspired him to create this easy-drinking saison. It benefits from warmer fermentation temperatures, and he ramps it up from 68°F (20°C) to the middle to upper 70s Fahrenheit (24–26°C) over the course of a few days. It can take a long time for beer to develop Brett character. It also has the tendency to attenuate slowly, which is something to be mindful of when packaging! Don't rush into bottling or kegging until you are certain that there is zero fermentation, so you don't inadvertently create bottle bombs. Stuart recommends reading *American Sour Beers* by Michael Tonsmeire and getting to know the Milk the Funk community online for more information on successfully making Brett beers (http://www.milkthefunk.com/wiki/).

For 5 US gal. (18.9 L)

Original gravity: 1.054 (13.3°P)
Final gravity: 1.005 (1.3°P)
Color: 5 SRM (10 EBC)

IBU: 30
ABV: 6.44%

FERMENTABLES
5.75 lb. (2.61 kg) Grouse pale millet malt
2.25 lb. (1.02 kg) Grouse Vienna millet malt
1.50 lb. (0.68 kg) Eckert biscuit rice malt
1.00 lb. (0.45 kg) Grouse buckwheat malt

0.25 lb. (0.11 kg) Grouse Cara Millet malt
1.00 lb. (0.45 kg) Bob's Red Mill® raw unmalted millet

ENZYMES
12 mL Ondea® Pro (equivalent to 0.98 mL/lb. grain, or 2.16 mL/kg)
15 mL Ceremix® Flex (1.2 mL/lb. grain, or 2.7 mL/kg)

WATER
Ca^{2+}: 80 ppm, Mg^{2+}: 5 ppm, Na^+: 25 ppm, Cl^-: 75 ppm, SO_4^{2-}: 80 ppm, HCO_3^-: 100 ppm

HOPS
1 oz. (28 g) East Kent Goldings (5% AA) @ 45 min.
1 oz. (28 g) Tettnanger (4.5% AA) @ 15 min.
1 oz. (28 g) Saaz (3.5% AA) @ 5 min.

ADDITIONAL INGREDIENTS
small pinch Irish moss @ 15 min.
0.08 oz. (2.3 g) Yeastex 61 yeast nutrient (allergen warning: contains soy) @ 15 min.

YEAST
Propagate Lab Farmhouse MIP-300, or other saison strain such as LalBrew Farmhouse™
Additional yeast: Propagate Lab Brett Brux I MIP-701, or SafBrew™ BR-8 (or any *Brettanomyces* strain you can find on gluten-free media)

Continued >

BREWING NOTES

1. Heat 4.0 gal. (15.1 L) strike water to 120°F (49°C; a liquor to grist ratio of 1.4 qt./lb.), mash in grains to achieve a rest temperature of 113°F (45°C), and rest for 10 min. (This serves as a quasi-ferulic acid rest.)
2. Raise mash to 125°F (52°C) and rest for 10 min.
3. Raise mash to 145°F (63°C) and rest for 60 min.
4. Raise mash to 175°F (79°C) and rest for 30 min.
5. Raise temperature to 180°F (82°C) and begin vorlauf.
6. Sparge using 175°F (79°C) water. Sparge until 6 gal. (22.7 L) of wort is collected in the boil kettle.
7. Boil for 60 minutes with hops, adding hops per schedule. Add a pinch of Irish moss and Yeastex 61 yeast nutrient with 15 min. left in the boil.
8. Once boil is finished, chill the wort to 75°F (24°C) and pitch yeast. Note that Brett can be co-pitched or added later for different results.
9. Ferment at 68°F (20°C). Once terminal gravity has been reached, cold crash until the beer is clear of suspended yeast.
10. Package and carbonate to 2.8 vol. CO_2. **Take care:** check the manufacturer's specification to ensure that your bottles can withstand higher levels of carbonation and avoid exploding bottles. Err on the side of caution since some standard beer bottles are not rated for high levels of carbonation and may explode.

FLANDERS BROWN SOUR
Gluten-Free Oud Bruin
Contributed by Stuart Cole

Oud bruin is a Belgian beer style that marries sour and malty flavors that evoke dark fruits like raisin and fig. The darker malts and candi syrup in this recipe are there for a bit of color, to accentuate those dried fruit flavors, and to provide just a hint of roast. Though maybe a little less complex than traditional mixed culture sours, the kettle sour approach works fine for a quick turnaround, allowing you to dial in the level of acidity before boiling to halt the process. An alternative approach would be to use a hybrid lactic acid-producing yeast like Lallemand's WildBrew™ Philly Sour (a species of the genus *Lachancea*).

For 5 US gal. (18.9 L)

Original gravity: 1.065 (15.9°P)
Final gravity: 1.010 (2.6°P)
Color: 33 SRM (65 EBC)

IBU: 0
ABV: 7.3%

FERMENTABLES
4.00 lb. (1.81 kg) Grouse pale millet malt
2.00 lb. (0.91 kg) Grouse Munich millet malt
1.00 lb. (0.45 kg) Grouse Cara Millet malt
1.00 lb. (0.45 kg) Grouse pale buckwheat malt
1.00 lb. (0.45 kg) Grouse raw unmalted millet
0.50 lb. (0.23 kg) Grouse Dutch Roast millet malt
0.50 lb. (0.23 kg) Eckert de-hulled "Gas Hog" rice malt

0.25 lb. (0.11 kg) Grouse Caramel 240L millet malt
1.00 lb. (0.45 kg) dried figs
1.00 lb. (0.45 kg) Candi Syrup, Inc. D-180™ dark candi syrup

ENZYMES
10 mL Ondea® Pro (equivalent to 0.98 mL/lb. grain, or 2.15 mL/kg)
15 mL Ceremix® Flex (1.46 mL/lb. grain, or 3.22 mL/kg)

WATER
Ca^{2+}: 43 ppm, Mg^{2+}: 24 ppm, Na^+: 38 ppm, Cl^-: 62 ppm, SO_4^{2-}: 66 ppm, HCO_3^-: 141 ppm

HOPS
2 oz. (57 g) US Tettnanger (3% AA) @ dry hop for 2 days

YEAST AND BACTERIA
If kettle souring:
- Lallemand WildBrew™ Sour Pitch (*Lactobacillus plantarum*) or an alternative lactic acid bacteria
- Fermentis SafAle™ US-05, or Fermentis SafAle™ K-97

Alternative single pitch and fermentation:
- Lallemand WildBrew™ Philly Sour (*Lachancea* spp.)

BREWING NOTES
1. Perform a rising-step mash. Mash in using 4.5 gal. (17 L) strike water, add Ondea Pro and Ceremix Flex enzymes, and rest at 125°F (52°C) for 15 min.
2. Raise mash temperature to 145°F (63°C) and rest for 60 min. Raise mash temperature to 175°F (79°C) and rest for a further 60 min.

Continued >

3. Before the mash is finished, preheat 1.5 gal. (5.7 L) sparge water to 175°F (79°C). At the end of the mash, perform your sparge to collect a pre-boil volume of approximately 6 gal. (22.7 L).

4. Boil the wort for 45 min. Do not add hops to the boil if kettle souring as this will inhibit the lactic acid bacteria. Proceed to step 5 if kettle souring, **or** proceed to step 6 if using a single pitch of Lallemand WildBrew Philly Sour.

5. Kettle sour: Leave boiled wort in the kettle. Pre-acidify wort to pH 4.2 before adding lactic acid bacteria. This will reduce risk of contamination by other bacteria and may improve eventual foam formation once packaged.

   a. Pitch the WildBrew™ Sour Pitch (or your lactic acid bacteria of choice) into 100°F (38°C), pre-acidified wort. Add some CO_2 to the kettle headspace before covering with a lid.

   b. Keep the inoculated wort at 100°F (38°C) for 12–25 hours, checking the pH and tasting as the lactic acid bacteria goes to work. Aim for an acidity level of about pH 3.2–3.5.

   c. When your desired acidity is reached, bring the wort to a boil and boil for 60 min. Chop up the dried figs and reconstitute with wort from kettle. Add figs and candi syrup to the last 10 minutes of boil.

   d. Cool wort to 68–70°F (20–21°C) and transfer to a fermentor. Pitch the ale yeast (US-05 or K-97) and ferment for 14 days at 80°F (27°C).

   e. Proceed to step 7.

6. Single pitch of Philly Sour: Before the boil is over, chop up the dried figs and reconstitute with hot wort from the kettle. Add to the last 10 minutes of the boil. Once the boil is finished, cool the wort to 75°F (24°C) and transfer to the fermentor. Pitch the WildBrew Philly Sour yeast and ferment at 75°F (24°C) for 30 days. Proceed to step 7.

7. Dry hop beer for 2 days before packaging. Carbonate to 2.8 vol. CO_2. **Take care:** check the manufacturer's specification to ensure that your bottles can withstand higher levels of carbonation and avoid exploding bottles. Err on the side of caution since some standard beer bottles are not rated for high levels of carbonation and may explode.

FARMHOUSE SAISON
Gluten-Free Classic Saison

Contributed by Jason Yerger of Mutantis Brewing, Portland, OR

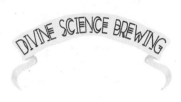

This recipe leaves a lot of room for improvisation—you don't really need to stick with basil and oak, you can try a range of herbs and spices as well as a variety of woods to age it on. Pink peppercorn, elderflower, or even Sichuan pepper would be good flavors to choose; if you can get your hands on cedar or ash, those would make nice woods for aging. Basil and oak do make a fine combination though! The grain bill emphasizes lighter rice malts, which encourages the production of esters and phenols when fermented with Belgian yeast. Buckwheat malt and caramel millet malt are great for promoting head retention without adding too much color, and demerara sugar helps keep the body light and crisp, as a saison should be.

For 5 US gal. (18.9 L)

Original gravity: 1.063 (15.4°P)
Final gravity: 1.009 (2.3°P)
Color: 6 SRM (12 EBC)

IBU: 19
ABV: 7.3%

FERMENTABLES
4.0 lb. (1.81 kg) Grouse pale buckwheat malt
4.0 lb. (1.81 kg) Eckert pale rice malt
2.0 lb. (0.91 kg) Eckert biscuit rice malt (4°L)
1.0 lb. (0.45 kg) Grouse Vienna millet malt
1.0 lb. (0.45 kg) Grouse caramel millet malt
0.5 lb. (0.23 kg) demerara sugar or dextrose (add at start of boil)

ENZYMES
10 mL Termamyl® SC DS (equivalent to 0.8 mL/lb. grain, or 1.8 mL/kg)
12 mL Ceremix® Flex (1 mL/lb. grain, or 2.2 mL/kg)
14 mL Ondea® Pro (1.2 mL/lb. grain, or 2.6 mL/kg)

WATER
Ca^{2+}: 46 ppm, Mg^{2+}: 11 ppm, Na^+: 3 ppm, SO_4^{2-}: 76 ppm, Cl^-: 61 ppm, HCO_3^-: 0 ppm

HOPS
1.6 oz. (45 g) Crystal (3.5% AA) @ 60 min.

ADDITIONAL INGREDIENTS
1 oz. (28 g) fresh basil @ 10 min.
1 tablet Whirlfloc @ 10 min.
3 oz. (85 g) French oak cubes @ secondary fermentor

YEAST
1 sachet (11.5 g, or 0.4 oz.) Fermentis SafAle™ T-58

BREWING NOTES
1. Perform a rising-step mash. Mash in, add all three enzymes, and rest at 125°F (52°C) for 20 min.
2. Raise mash temperature to 145°F (63°C) over the course of 20 min., then hold for 45 min.
3. Raise mash temperature to 175°F (79°C) over the course of 20 min., then hold for 30 min.

Continued >

4. Before the mash is finished, preheat sparge water to 209°F (98°C). At the end of the mash, perform your sparge to collect a pre-boil volume of approximately 6 gal. (22.7 L).
5. Boil for 60 min., adding sugar/dextrose, hops, basil, and Whirlfloc as scheduled.
6. When the boil is complete, cool the wort to 78°F (26°C) and transfer to the fermentor. Pitch yeast and ferment at 78°F (26°C) for 14 days.
7. Transfer to secondary vessel and cold condition on oak cubes for 21 days at 38°F (3°C).
8. Package and serve. Carbonate to 2.8 vol. CO_2. **Take care:** check the manufacturer's specification to ensure that your bottles can withstand higher levels of carbonation and avoid exploding bottles. Err on the side of caution since some standard beer bottles are not rated for high levels of carbonation and may explode.

SWEET POTATOES & RICE & BELGIAN SPICE
Gluten-Free Belgian Spiced Ale
Contributed by Robert Keifer

During the COVID-19 shutdown, I had a lot more time at home to do things like gardening, which has become a true joy in my life. One of the crops that I was able to farm well in my apartment complex was sweet potato—one plant must have returned north of 20 pounds of sweet potatoes! I decided to eat half and brew with the other half. Harvest time for this plant was around September, which is also very close to pumpkin spice/holiday season. One of my favorite things to enjoy in the fall is sweet potato pie, so that really became a huge influence on this recipe in terms of the spice additions and choosing a yeast known for eliciting fruity and spicy flavors.

For 5.5 US gal. (20.8 L)

Original gravity: 1.042 (10.5°P)
Final gravity: 1.011 (2.8°P)
Color: 15 SRM (30 EBC)

IBU: 12
ABV: 4.1%

FERMENTABLES
10 lb. (4.54 kg) sweet potato, grated
5 lb. (2.27 kg) Eckert crystal rice

ENZYMES
11 mL Termamyl® SC DS (equivalent to 0.7 mL/lb. fermentables, or 1.6 mL/kg)
25 mL SEBAmyl® L (1.7 mL/lb. fermentables, or 3.7 mL/kg)

WATER
Ca^{2+}: 66 ppm, Mg^{2+}: 26 ppm, Na^+: 96 ppm Cl^-: 94 ppm, SO_4^{2-}: 216 ppm, HCO_3^-: 209 ppm

HOPS
1 oz. (28 g) Hallertauer Mittelfrüher (3.7% AA) @ 60 min.

ADDITIONAL INGREDIENTS
¾ tsp. (3 g) grains of paradise, ground @ 15 min.
1 tsp. (4 g) nutmeg, ground @ 15 min.

YEAST
1 sachet (11.5 g, or 0.4 oz.) Fermentis SafAle™ T-58

BREWING NOTES
1. Perform a reverse or falling temperature step mash. Mash in the rice first using 3 gal. (11.4 L) strike water heated to 205°F (96°C) to achieve a mash temperature of 190°F (87°C). Add the Termamyl SC DS and rest at 190°F (88°C) for 20 min.
2. Mash in the sweet potato to reach 170°F (77°C), adding cold or room-temperature water if necessary to drop the temperature. Rest for an additional 30 min.
3. Allow to cool to 150°F (65.5°C) and add SEBAmyl L. Rest for 20 mins.
4. Vorlauf until wort is clear. Sparge using 170°F (77°C) water.
5. Boil for 60 min., adding hops and spices as directed. Once the boil is finished, chill wort to 67°F (19°C).
6. Pitch yeast at 67°F (19°C) and let free rise without temperature control.
7. Once terminal gravity is reached, cold crash for up to 2 weeks until beer is clear. Carbonate to 2.7 volumes CO_2.

MOSAIC SAISON
Gluten-Free Hoppy Saison

Contributed by Ben Acord

This beer is inspired by Anchorage Brewing Company's Mosaic Saison—one of the most complex beers Ben had ever tasted. Head brewer, Gabe Fletcher, told Ben to try to push the boundaries of gluten free to the limit after Ben told him he was transitioning to gluten-free brewing. Gabe encouraged him to break away from tradition, which was reflected in Ben's prior brewing of high-gravity barrel-aged beers, as well as the wild/mixed-culture beers. This recipe is good base for your imagination. On its own, it is a hop forward saison. If you decide to add in other cultures of bacteria or yeast, the beer goes from good to great. Even bottles that are 4 or 5 years old are still bright, complex, and beautifully effervescent.

For 5.5 US gal. (20.8L)

Original gravity: 1.098 (12.8°P)
Final gravity: 1.006 (1.5°P)
Color: 2-6 SRM

IBU: 15-20
ABV: 12%

FERMENTABLES

13.0 lb. (5.90 kg) pale millet malt
1.5 lb. (0.68 kg) Vienna millet malt

1.5 lb. (0.68 kg) Munich millet malt
1.0 lb. (0.45 kg) unmalted millet malt

Optional: Clear Belgian candi syrup can be used to boost the gravity during fermentation, which will increase the final ABV and stress the yeast; as a wort booster, it can serve as a backup on brew day in case you undershoot your target original gravity.

ENZYMES

17 mL Termamyl® SC DS (equivalent to 1 mL/lb. grain, or 2.2 mL/kg)
34 mL SEBAmyl® L (2 mL/lb. grain, or 4.4 mL/kg)

WATER

Pilsen-style profile—soft water, very little salts

HOPS

2 oz. (57 g) Mosaic @ 5 min.

ADDITIONAL ITEMS

0.7 oz. (20 g) preferred yeast nutrient @ 15 min.
0.35 oz. (10 g) Irish moss @ 15 min.

YEASTS

6 g (½ sachet) Fermentis SafAle™ BE-134
6 g (½ sachet) Lallemand LalBrew® Farmhouse™
6 g (½ sachet) Lallemand LalBrew® Voss™- Kveik, for bottle conditioning (optional)

BREWING NOTES

1. Mash for 35 min. at 158°F (70°C) with Termamyl SC DS.
2. Mash for 45 min. at 145°F (63°C) with SEBAmyl L.
3. Sparge with 165°F (74°C) until 7 gal. (26.5 L) pre-boil wort is collected in kettle.
4. Boil wort for 60 min., adding kettle/whirlpool hops as indicated.
5. Once boil is finished, chill wort to 68°F (20°C) and pitch yeast

6. Ferment at 68°F (20°C) until specific gravity is about half the original gravity. Then let temperature free rise.

7. Once specific gravity is close to finishing gravity, lower the temperature to 58°F (14°C) and let sit for 3 days.

8. Kegging: Rack into secondary and let sit for 3–4 weeks between 38°F (3°C) and 50°F (10°C), then transfer and carbonate in keg.

9. Bottling: Bottle condition with Lallemand Lalbrew Voss and clear Belgian candi syrup in champagne bottles to 2.7–3.0 vols CO_2. Candi Syrup, Inc. has a helpful reference called "Priming with Candi Syrups" that can help (https://www.candisyrup.com/help-docs.html). **Take care:** check the manufacturer's specification to ensure that your bottles can withstand higher levels of carbonation and avoid exploding bottles. Err on the side of caution since some standard beer bottles are not rated for high levels of carbonation and may explode.

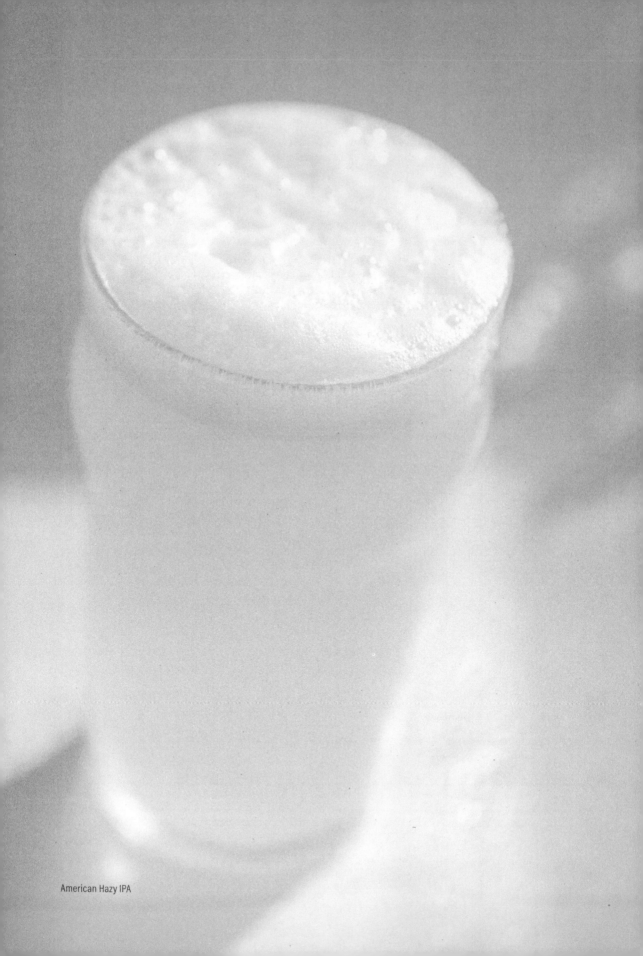

American Hazy IPA

9

Modern New World Beers

Taken from modern-day American craft beer offerings, the following beer recipes are inspired by brewers who have pushed the limits. From playful to downright scientific, there are some truly interesting flavor profiles available to the modern gluten-free brewer.

JAMES BLONDE
Gluten-Free American Blonde Ale

Contributed by Bierly Brewing, McMinnville, OR

Bierly Brewing's head brewer, JP (p. 111) used the James Blonde recipe to experiment with different mash regimes before arriving at the three-step rising mash regime you see here. Subtle expressions of bread-like sweetness, grainy textures, and lemony hop notes can be coaxed out of this recipe depending on how you run your mash. The results are best with the three-step rising mash, but this recipe turns out well with other mash regimes; try using a single-step infusion mash or the falling temperature mash. Playing with low-IBU beers like James Blonde allows you to discover just how complex the flavors of gluten-free malts can be.

For 5 US gal. (18.9 L)

Original gravity: 1.055 (13.6°P)
Final gravity: 1.012 (3.1°P)
Color: 8 SRM (16 EBC)

IBU: 23
ABV: 5.6%

GRAIN BILL
7.25 lb. (3.29 kg) Grouse pale millet malt
2.50 lb. (1.13 kg) Eckert crystal rice malt

2.25 lb. (1.02 kg) Eckert pale rice malt
0.35 lb. (0.16 kg) Grouse Munich millet malt

ENZYMES
12 mL Ceremix® Flex (equivalent to 0.97 mL/lb. grain, or 2.14 mL/kg)
12 mL Termamyl® SC DS (0.97 mL/lb. grain, or 2.14 mL/kg)
12 mL Ondea® Pro (0.97 mL/lb. grain, or 2.14 mL/kg)

WATER
Based on McMinnville, OR water profile:
Ca^{2+}: 9 ppm, Mg^{2+}: 2 ppm, Na^+: 8 ppm, Cl^-: 6 ppm, SO_4^{2-}: 9 ppm, Alkalinity (as $CaCO_3$): 19 ppm, pH: 7.28

HOPS
1.25 oz. (35 g) Crystal (3.6% AA) @ 60 min.
0.75 oz. (21 g) Crystal (3.6% AA) @ 10 min.
0.75 oz. (21 g) Crystal (3.6% AA) @ whirlpool for 20 min.

ADDITIONAL INGREDIENTS
small pinch Irish moss @ 15 min.
0.08 oz. (2.3 g) Yeastex 61 yeast nutrient (allergen warning: contains soy) @ 15 min.

YEAST
1 sachet (11.5 g, or 0.4 oz.) Fermentis SafAle™ S-04

BREWING NOTES
1. Perform a rising-step mash. Mash in using 4.5 gal. (17 L) strike water, add all three enzymes, and rest at 125°F (52°C) for 20 min. Mash pH should come in at 5.2–5.3.
2. Raise mash temperature to 145°F (63°C) and rest for 45 min. Raise mash temperature to 175°F (79°C) and rest for 20 min.
3. Before the mash is finished, preheat sparge water to 209°F (98°C). At the end of the mash, perform your sparge to collect a pre-boil volume of approximately 6.5 gal. (24.6 L).
4. When the boil is complete, cool the wort to 68°F (20°C) and transfer to the fermentor.
5. Pitch yeast and ferment at 68°F (20°C) for 14 days.
6. Cold crash beer until the liquid is clear. Carbonate to 2.5 vol. CO_2.

4-GRAIN CREAM ALE
Gluten-Free American Cream Ale

Contributed by Jason Yerger of Mutantis Brewing, Portland, OR

Cream ale is a great style for brewing gluten free, as the style typically incorporates some amount of corn and/or rice even when brewed with barley. In this recipe, rice features prominently. Eckert's biscuit rice malt kilned to 4°L ("light biscuit") is one of my favorite base malts, as it has a light mild flavor but tastes more cereal-like than pale rice malt (which to me, tastes more like honey than a malt). Malted corn (maize) in this recipe adds a surprising amount of body and head retention, as well as a gentle fruitiness; you could even swap the quantities between the malted corn and the malted millet to get better head and a grainier flavor. Flaked quinoa also helps a bit with head retention and dries out the beer a little bit, in my experience.

For 5 US gallons (18.9 L)

Original gravity: 1.044 (11.0°P)
Final gravity: 1.012 (3.1°P)
Color: 4 SRM (9 EBC)

IBU: 15
ABV: 4.1%

FERMENTABLES
3.0 lb. (1.36 kg) Grouse pale malted millet
4.0 lb. (1.81 kg) Eckert biscuit rice malt 4°L

1.0 lb. (0.45 kg) Grouse malted yellow corn
1.0 lb. (0.45 kg) Grouse flaked quinoa

ENZYMES
9 mL Termamyl® SC DS (equivalent to 1.0 mL/lb. grain, or 2.2 mL/kg)
9 mL Ceremix® Flex (1.0 mL/lb. grain, or 2.2 mL/kg)
11 mL Ondea® Pro (1.2 mL/lb. grain, or 2.7 mL/kg)

WATER
Ca^{2+}: 50 ppm, Mg^{2+}: 9.5 ppm, Na^+: 5 ppm, SO_4^{2-}: 105 ppm, Cl^-: 45 ppm, HCO_3^-: 0 ppm

HOPS
0.2 oz. (6 g) Sterling (7.5% AA) @ 5 min.

ADDITIONAL ITEMS
1 tablet Whirlfloc @ 10 min.

YEAST
1 sachet (11 g, or 0.39 oz.) Lallemand LalBrew BRY-97™

BREWING NOTES
1. Perform a rising-step mash. Mash in using 4 gal. (15 L) strike water, add all three enzymes, and rest at 125°F (52°C) for 20 min.
2. Raise mash temperature to 155°F (68°C) over the course of 20 min., then hold for 45 min.
3. Raise mash temperature to 175°F (79°C) over the course of 20 min., then hold for 30 min.
4. Before the mash is finished, preheat sparge water to 209°F (98°C). At the end of the mash, perform your sparge to collect a pre-boil volume of approximately 6 gal. (22.7 L).
5. Boil for 60 min., adding hops and Whirlfloc as scheduled.
6. When the boil is complete, cool the wort and transfer to the fermentor. Pitch yeast and ferment at 65°F (18°C) for 14 days.
7. Cold condition 5 days at 38°F (3°C).
8. Package and serve. Carbonate to 2.4 vol. CO_2.

INCLUSION PALE ALE
Gluten-Free American Pale Ale

Contributed by Ground Breaker Brewing, Portland, OR

Ground Breaker Brewing opened its doors in 2011 believing that anyone should be able to participate in craft beer culture that wanted to. Its first beer was a pale ale, brewed to be accessible and tasty to as broad an audience of craft beer enthusiasts as possible. Ground Breaker has improved on the recipe, but the spirit and principles on which the brewery and brand was founded haven't changed. Craft beer is all about inclusion at Ground Breaker.

For 5 US gal. (18.9 L)

Original gravity: 1.057 Plato: (14°P)
Final gravity: 1.010 (2.6°P)
Color: 5 SRM (9 EBC)

IBU: 29
ABV: 6.1%

FERMENTABLES
1.05 lb. (0.48 kg) Eckert pale rice malt
0.70 lb. (0.32 kg) Eckert biscuit rice malt 4°L
0.50 lb. (0.23 kg) Grouse pale buckwheat malt
0.50 lb. (0.23 kg) flaked quinoa
0.35 lb. (0.16 kg) amber rice malt 15°L
4.80 lb. (2.18 kg) BriesSweet™ White Sorghum Extract – to be added before boil

0.50 lb. (0.23 kg) organic tapioca maltodextrin – to be added before boil
0.50 lb. (0.23 kg) cane sugar – to be added before boil

ENZYMES
4 mL Ceremix® Flex (1.3 mL/lb. of grain in mash, or 2.9 mL/kg)

HOPS
0.36 oz. (10 g) Nugget (12.5% AA) @ 60 min.
0.40 oz. (11 g) Cascade (9.2% AA) @ 15 min.
0.16 oz. (5 g) Meridian (5.7% AA) @ 1 min.
0.28 oz. (8 g) Cascade (9.2% AA) @ 1 min.
0.48 oz. (14 g) Cascade (9.2% AA) @ dry hop for 3 days
0.48 oz. (14 g) Meridian (5.7% AA) @ dry hop for 3 days

ADDITIONAL ITEMS
½ tablet Whirfloc @ 15 min.
1 oz. (28 g) diammonium phosphate (DAP) yeast nutrient @ 15 min.

YEAST
1 package (11.5 oz., or 0.4 oz.) Fermentis SafAle™ US-05

BREWING NOTES
1. Perform a single-infusion mash, using Ceremix Flex at 1.323 mL/lb. of grain (2.917 mL/kg) per manufacturer's recommendation, not counting the syrup, sugar, and maltodextrin.
2. Mash in to achieve mash temperature of 163°F (73°C), add enzyme, and hold for 90 min.
3. Vorlauf for 15 min. and transfer to the kettle. Add the sorghum syrup, maltodextrin, and cane sugar once wort is transferred to the kettle (without flame to prevent scorching).
4. Boil wort for 60 min., adding hops, Whirfloc, and nutrients according to schedule.
5. Once the boil is finished, cool wort to 68°F (20°C).
6. Pitch yeast and ferment at 68°F (20°C) for 2 weeks.
7. Cold crash for 3 days and package. Carbonate to 2.5 vol. CO_2.

CHICO PALE ALE
Gluten-Free American Pale Ale

Contributed by Robert Keifer

I grew up in Northern California and my first craft beer experience was Sierra Nevada Pale Ale. When I think of pale ale (yes, some British ales that I have tried come to mind) I always compare them to Sierra Nevada Pale Ale. It took about 20 iterations of this recipe and process to dial it in. I can honestly say, this is about as close as I've been able to come to being able to clone Sierra Nevada Pale Ale's unique taste that has never let me down.

For 5 U.S. gallons (18.9 L)

Original gravity: 1.058 (14.3°P)　　　　　**IBU:** 40
Final gravity: 1.016 (4.1°P)　　　　　**ABV:** 5.5%
Color: 9–10 SRM (18–20 EBC)

FERMENTABLES

3.0 lb. (1.36 kg) Eckert de-hulled pale rice malt　　1.5 lb. (0.68 kg) Grouse pale buckwheat malt
5.0 lb. (2.27 kg) Eckert biscuit rice 5°L　　0.5 lb. (0.23 kg) Grouse Dutch Roast millet malt
1.5 lb. (0.68 kg) Grouse Vienna millet malt　　0.5 lb. (0.23 kg) Grouse roasted Cara Millet malt

ENZYMES

12.25 mL Termamyl® SC DS (equivalent to 1.02 mL/lb. grain, or 2.25 mL/kg)
15 mL SEBAmyl® L (1.25 mL/lb. grain, or 2.75 mL/kg)

HOPS

1 oz. (28 g) Cascade (6.5% AA) @ 60 min.
1 oz. (28 g) Cascade (6.5% AA) @ whirlpool for 20 min., 180°F (82°C)
1 oz. (28 g) Cascade (6.5% AA) dry hop (3 days before cold crash)

YEAST

1 package (11.5 g, 0.4 oz.) Fermentis SafAle™ S-04

BREWING NOTES

1. Heat 22.05 qt. (20.87 L) strike water and mash in with all grains to achieve a mash temperature of 195°F (91°C). Add Termamyl SC DS and rest for 20 min.
2. Recirculate mash liquid to lower the temperature or add 1.0 gal (3.79 L) of room-temperature water to the mash to bring the temperature down to 155°F (68°C). Add SEBAmyl L and rest for 30 min.
3. Vorlauf until clear then transfer to the boil kettle.
4. Boil for 60 min., adding hops per schedule, then cool the wort to 68°F (20°C).
5. Pitch yeast and ferment for 2 weeks at 68°F (20°C). Once airlock action is one bubble every 30–45 seconds, dry hop with Cascade and let sit for 3–5 days.
6. Cold crash until beer is clear. For extra clarity, add Biofine® at time of cold conditioning.

ZERO TOLERANCE GF CALIBRATION PALE ALE

Gluten-Free American Pale Ale *Contributed by Stuart Cole with participation from Robert Keifer*

Stuart's idea behind this beer was to have a somewhat standardized all-grain recipe that gluten free brewers could make to "calibrate" their results—a baseline for comparing the impact of different types of equipment, enzymes, and mash routines. The goal was to keep the fermentables list relatively simple and accessible to many (though recognizing that access to malted rice and millet varies around the world). A pale ale with a fairly restrained hop schedule and fermented with the widely available and fairly predictable US-05 "Chico" yeast.

When first introduced on the Zero Tolerance group Facebook page in 2020, Ondea Pro and Ceremix Flex enzymes were a popular combination, but this could be made with Ceremix Flex alone using a simple infusion mash or, of course, another combination of enzymes with potentially different extract and attenuation results. An alternative combination has been suggested below.

I did this same recipe with a falling step-mash that consisted of Termamyl SC DS and Sebamyl L and achieved very similar results (OG: 1.044, FG: 1.010; I used the Chico yeast from Cellar Science instead of Fermentis US-05).

For 5 US gal. (18.9 L)

Original Gravity: 1.045 (11.2°P)   **IBU:** 39
Final Gravity: 1.008 (2.1°C)   **ABV:** 4.9%
Color: 5 SRM (10 EBC)

FERMENTABLES
4.0 lb. (1.81 kg) Grouse pale millet malt   4.0 lb. (1.81 kg) Eckert biscuit rice malt 5°L
1.0 lb. (0.45 kg) Grouse Vienna millet malt

ENZYMES
Option 1:
    10 mL Ondea® Pro (equivalent to 1.1 mL/lb. grain, or 2.4 mL/kg)
    15 mL Ceremix® Flex (1.7 mL/lb. grain, or 3.7 mL/kg)
Option 2:
    10 mL Termamyl® SC DS (1.1 mL/lb. grain, or 2.4 mL/kg)
    20 mL SEBAmyl® L (2.2 mL/lb. grain, or 4.2 mL/kg)

HOPS
1.0 oz. (28 g) Cascade (7% AA) @ 25 min.
1.0 oz. (28 g) Cascade (7% AA) @ 10 min.
0.5 oz. (14 g) Amarillo (8.6% AA) @ 5 min.
1.0 oz. (28 g) Centennial (10% AA) @ 5 min.
0.5 oz. (14 g) Amarillo (8.6% AA) @ whirlpool at 170°F (77°C)
1.0 oz. (28 g) Centennial (10% AA) @ dry hop for 3 days

ADDITIONAL ITEMS
1 tablet Whirlfloc® @ 15 min.
0.08 oz. (2.3 g) Yeastex 61 yeast nutrient (allergen warning: contains soy) @ 15 min.

YEAST
1 package (11.5 g, or 0.4 oz.) Fermentis SafAle™ US-05

BREWING NOTES
1. Perform a rising step mash using the Ondea Pro, Ceremix Flex, and Termamyl SC DS.
2. Mash in using 4.5–5.0 gal. (17–19 L) strike water, add all three enzymes, and rest at 125°F (52°C) for 20 min. Mash pH should come in at 5.2–5.3.
3. Raise mash temperature to 145°F (63°C) and rest for 45 min. Raise mash temperature to 175°F (79°C) and rest for 20 min.
4. Before the mash is finished, preheat sparge water to 180°F (82°C). At the end of the mash, perform your sparge to collect a pre-boil volume of approximately 6 gal. (22.7 L).
5. Boil for 60 min., adding hops, Whirlfloc, and yeast nutrient as scheduled.
6. When the boil and whirlpool are complete, cool the wort to 68°F (20°C) and transfer to the fermentor.
7. Ferment at 68°F (20°C) for up to 14 days. At the end of fermentation, add dry hops.
8. Cold age the beer for an additional 3–5 days, or until the liquid is clear.
9. Carbonate to 2.5 vol. CO_2.

EASY DOES IT PALE ALE
Gluten-Free West Coast American Pale Ale

Contributed by Aaron Gervais, Otherwise Brewing

The straightforward, single-infusion mash in this recipe lets you brew a tasty, everyday pale ale in the West Coast style without breaking your brain on complicated infusion calculations and multiple enzyme additions. Just mix everything up, wait 90 minutes, then drain to the kettle and boil! Sometimes simple is best.

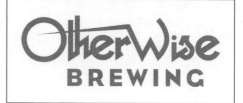

For 6 US gal. (22.7 L)

Original gravity: 1.051 (12.6°P)
Final gravity: 1.013 (3.3°P)
Color: 6 SRM (12 EBC)

IBU: 50
ABV: 5.0%

FERMENTABLES
12.00 lb. (5.44 kg) Eckert biscuit rice malt 4°L
0.75 lb. (0.34 kg) Eckert crystal rice malt

ENZYMES
9 mL Ceremix® Flex (equivalent to 0.7 mL/lb. grain, or 1.6 mL/kg)
5 mL Termamyl® (0.4 mL/lb. grain, or 0.9 mL/kg)

HOPS
0.5 oz. (14 g) CTZ (15% AA) @ 60 min.
0.5 oz. (14 g) CTZ (15% AA) @ 10 min.
1.0 oz. (28 g) Cascade (7% AA) @ 10min.
3.0 oz. (85 g) Cascade (7% AA) @ whirlpool/hop stand for 15 min.

YEAST
1 sachet (11.0–11.5 g, or 0.39–0.4 oz.) American or British ale yeast of choice

BREWING NOTES
1. Mash into 19.13 qt. (18.1 L) of 190°F (88°C) hot water. Once mash temperature is down to 180°F (82°C), add enzymes and rest for 90 min. at 175°F (79°C).
2. Sparge with 2.5 gal. (9.5 L) of 209°F (98°C) hot water, collecting 7.0 gal. (26.5 L) in the boil kettle.
3. Boil for 60 min. Once boil and whirlpool/hop stand are complete, chill wort to 68°F (20°C).
4. Pitch yeast and ferment at 68°F (20°C) for 2 weeks, or until terminal gravity is reached.
5. Cold crash until beer is clear, and carbonate to 2.5 vol. CO_2.

GHOST IN THE FOG
Gluten-Free American Hazy IPA

From Brian Newcomb, Troy, MI

Brian is doubly invested in gluten-free brewing: he is owner of Gluten Free Brew Supply gfbsupply.com) and an avid homebrewer. This is his recipe for a gluten-free New England-style IPA. The beer is silky and hazy from the use of oats, and the fruitiness from the sorghum malt. I can attest to the incredibly silky mouthfeel and spooky great taste!

For 5.5 gal. (20.8 L)

Original gravity: 1.056 (13.8°P)
Final gravity: 1.006 (1.3°P)
Color: 5 SRM (11 EBC)

IBU: 52
ABV: 6.6%

FERMENTABLES

7.0 lb. (3.18 kg) red sorghum malt
4.0 lb. (1.81 kg) oat malt

1.0 lb. (0.45 kg) buckwheat malt

ENZYMES

12 mL Ceremix® Flex (equivalent to 1.0 mL/lb. grain, or 2.2 mL/kg)
12 mL Termamyl® SC DS (1.0 mL/lb. grain, or 2.2 mL/kg)
12 mL Ondea® Pro (1.0 mL/lb. grain, or 2.2 mL/kg)

HOPS

0.5 oz. (14 g) Centennial (10.5% AA) @ 60 min.
1.0 oz. (28 g) Citra (12% AA) @ 10 min.
1.0 oz. (28 g) Centennial (10.5% AA) @ 10 min.
1.0 oz. (28 g) Amarillo (10% AA) @ whirlpool at 175° (79°C) for 15 min.
1.0 oz. (28 g) Citra (12% AA) @ whirlpool at 175° (79°C) for 15 min.
1.0 oz. (28 g) Amarillo (10% AA) @ dry hop – add on day 2 of fermentation
1.0 oz. (28 g) Citra (12% AA) @ dry hop – add when primary fermentation finished

YEAST

1 sachet (11 g) Lalbrew Voss™ – Kveik Ale Yeast

BREWING NOTES

1. Perform a rising-step mash. Mash in using 4.5 gal. (17 L) strike water, add all three enzymes, and rest at 125°F (52°C) for 20 min. Mash pH should come in at 5.2–5.3.
2. Raise mash temperature to 145°F (63°C) and rest for 45 min. Raise mash temperature to 175°F (79°C) and rest for 20 min.
3. Before the mash is finished, preheat sparge water to 180°F (82°C). At the end of the mash, perform your sparge to collect a pre-boil volume of approximately 6 gal. (22.7 L).
4. Boil wort for 60 min., adding hops according to schedule.
5. When the boil and whirlpool are complete, cool the wort to 68°F (20°C), transfer to the fermentor, and pitch yeast.
6. Let fermentation rise to 85°F (29°C) and ferment for 4 days, dry hopping with Amarillo hops on day 2 of active fermentation.
7. Dry hop with 1 oz. (28 g) Citra hops at the end of active fermentation for 24 hours.
8. Cold crash to drop hops and yeast out of suspension before packaging. Carbonate to 2.4 vol. CO_2.

FOOL'S GOLD NEIPA
Gluten-Free Hazy/Juicy IPA

Contributed by Ben Fowler

In 2016, Ben Fowler discovered that he was gluten intolerant. As a craft beer lover, Ben found it a struggle to accept that his options were limited to cider or wine. He took to the internet to find a way to home brew gluten-free beer. He discovered the Zero Tolerance Homebrew Club on Facebook and has been consumed by homebrewing ever since.

This beer was inspired by Ben's drinking friends who enjoy, almost exclusively, barley-based hazy IPAs. Something about the hazy, orange juice–colored beer always looked so refreshing in summer, so Ben had to create his own. He called this beer Fool's Gold because those same friends are unable to distinguish this beer from the barley-based hazies they drink on the regular.

For 5.5 gal. (20.8 L)

Original gravity: 1.071 (17.3°P)
Final gravity: 1.012 (3.1°P)
Color: 6 SRM (11 EBC)

IBU: 64
ABV: 7.9%

FERMENTABLES

8.0 lb. (3.63 kg) Grouse pale millet malt
3.5 lb. (1.59 kg) Grouse pale buckwheat malt
1.0 lb. (0.45 kg) Bob's Red Mill® Gluten Free Old Fashioned Rolled Oats (certified gluten free)
1.0 lb. (0.45 kg) Grouse Vienna millet malt

0.5 lb. (0.23 kg) Grouse caramel millet malt 4°L
0.5 lb. (0.23 kg) Grouse unmalted flaked quinoa
0.5 lb. (0.23 kg) Grouse Cara Millet malt
1.5 lb. (0.68 kg) rice hulls – to aid with wort separation

ENZYMES

15 mL Termamyl® SC DS (equivalent to 1.0 mL/lb. grain, or 2.2 mL/kg)
15 mL SEBAmyl® L (1.0 mL/lb. grain, or 2.2 mL/kg)
18 mL Ondea® Pro (1.2 mL/lb. grain, or 2.6 mL/kg)

HOPS

1.00 oz. (28 g) Citra (12% AA) @ 55 min.
1.00 oz. (28 g) Galaxy (14% AA) @ 55 min.
1.50 oz. (43 g) Citra (12% AA) @ whirlpool at 170°F (77°C) for 15 min.
1.50 oz. (43 g) Galaxy (14% AA) @ whirlpool at 170°F (77°C) for 15 min.
1.50 oz. (43 g) Mosaic (12.5% AA) @ whirlpool at 170°F (77°C) for 15 min.
1.00 oz. (28 g) Citra (12% AA) @ dry hop for 7 days – add at high krausen*
1.50 oz. (43 g) Citra (12% AA) @ dry hop for 7 days – add at high krausen
1.00 oz. (28 g) Mosaic (12.5% AA) @ dry hop for 7 days – add at high krausen
1.25 oz. (35 g) Citra (12% AA) @ dry hop for 3 days
1.50 oz. (43 g) Galaxy (14% AA) @ dry hop for 3 days
1.00 oz. (28 g) Mosaic (12.5% AA) @ dry hop for 3 days

* High krausen (*kräusen*) is a German brewing term for the vigorous and often unruly head of foam that foams atop a fermenting beer at the peak of fermentation.

ADDITIONAL ITEMS

4 tsp (10 g) Yeastex 61 yeast nutrient (allergen warning: contains soy) @ 15 min.
3 tsp (7 g) Irish moss @ 15 min.

YEAST

1 sachet (11.5 g) Propagate Lab's gluten-free hazy IPA yeast or any NEIPA dry yeast

BREWING NOTES

1. Add 22.89 qt. (21.66 L) strike water (liquor to grist ratio of 1.25 qt./lb.) and mash at 185°F (85°C) for 60 min. with the Termamyl SC DS.
2. Add 2–3 qt. (1.9–2.8 L) cold water until mash temperature drops to 145°F (63°C). Add the SEBAmyl L and Ondea Pro enzymes. Rest for 90 min.
3. Sparge with 209°F (98°C) water. Boil and hop as directed above.
4. Once the boil and whirlpool are finished, chill to 67°F (19°C).
5. Pitch yeast and ferment at 67°F (19°C) for 6 days.
6. Rack to secondary and cold crash. Keg and serve. Carbonate to 2.3 vol. CO_2.

HAZY IPA
Gluten-Free Hazy IPA

Contributed by Ken Orner

After years of brewing barley beers, Ken was diagnosed with celiac disease. He was also a brewer at a local brewery, so he immediately began taking precautions. Since Ken could no longer enjoy barley-based beer, he started researching alternative grains for making beer. He turned to the internet and came across Zero Tolerance Gluten Free Homebrewing Club. They had a plethora of information available. Ken began experimenting with the different grains and enzymes available to develop a hazy IPA so he could enjoy something similar to what he was brewing at work, finally coming up with the recipe below. This recipe was inspired by Trillium beers that he loved to drink. This beer also won third place in the alternative grain category (War Of the Worts 2021 Category 31a Bronze medal) and it was the only beer that was 100% alternative grain and gluten free.

For 4 US gal. (15.14 L)

Original gravity: 1.066 (16°P)
Final gravity: 1.010 (3°P)
Color: 7 SRM (13 EBC)

IBU: 28
ABV: 7.4%

FERMENTABLES
5.0 lb. (2.26 kg) Grouse pale millet malt
1.5 lb. (0.68 kg) Bob's Red Mill® Gluten Free Old Fashioned Rolled Oats (certified gluten free)
1.0 lb. (0.45 kg) Grouse Goldfinch millet malt

0.5 lb. (0.23 kg) Grouse flaked quinoa
0.5 lb. (0.23 kg) Eckert biscuit rice malt 4°L
0.5 lb. (0.23 kg) Bob's Red Mill® unmalted millet

ENZYMES
16 mL Ceremix® Flex (equivalent to 1.8 mL/lb. grain, or 3.9 mL/kg)
11 mL Ondea® Pro (1.2 mL/lb. grain, or 2.7 mL/kg)
2 mL SebAmyl® L (0.2 mL/lb. grain, or 0.5 mL/kg)
3.2 mL Termamyl® SC DS (0.4 mL/lb. grain, or 0.8 mL/kg)

WATER
Ca^{2+} 124 ppm, Mg^{2+} 13 ppm, Na^+ 16 ppm, SO_4^{2-} 224 ppm, Cl^- 15 ppm, HCO_3^- 21 ppm. Acidify sparge water to pH of 6.

BOIL AND WHIRLPOOL HOPS
0.75 oz. (21 g) Citra (12.0% AA) @ 60 min.
0.75 oz. (21 g) Mosaic (12.3% AA) @ whirlpool – 170°F (77°C)
0.75 oz. (21 g) Citra (12.0% AA) @ whirlpool – 170°F (77°C)
0.75 oz. (21 g) Galaxy (14% AA) @ whirlpool – 170°F (77°C)
0.75 oz. (21 g) El Dorado (15.0% AA) @ whirlpool – 170°F (77°C)
1.00 oz. (28 g) Mosaic (12.3% AA) @ whirlpool – 155°F (68°C)
1.00 oz. (28 g) Citra (12.0% AA) @ whirlpool – 155°F (68°C)
1.00 oz. (28 g) Galaxy (14% AA) @ whirlpool – 155°F (68°C)
1.00 oz. (28 g) El Dorado (15.0% AA) @ whirlpool – 155°F (68°C)

ADDITIONAL ITEMS
1.0 lb. (0.45 kg) maltodextrin (to be added during boil as a slurry)
1 tablet Whirlfloc @ 10 min.

DRY HOPS

1.0 oz. (28 g) Mosaic (12.3% AA) @ dry hop at high krausen*
1.0 oz. (28 g) Citra (12.0% AA) @ dry hop at high krausen
1.0 oz. (28 g) Galaxy (14% AA) @ dry hop at high krausen
1.0 oz. (28 g) El Dorado (15.0% AA) @ dry hop at high krausen
1.0 oz. (28 g) Mosaic (12.3% AA) @ dry hop at end of fermentation
1.0 oz. (28 g) Citra (12.0% AA) @ dry hop at end of fermentation
1.0 oz. (28 g) Galaxy (14% AA) @ dry hop at end of fermentation
1.0 oz. (28 g) El Dorado (15.0% AA) @ dry hop at end of fermentation

* High krausen (*kräusen*) is a German brewing term for the vigorous and often unruly head of foam that foams atop a fermenting beer at the peak of fermentation.

YEAST

1 bottle (125 mL) Propagate Labs MIP-120

BREWING NOTES

1. Mash in with all four enzymes for 30 min. at 125°F (52°C), 60 min. at 145°F (63°C), 45 min. at 185°F (85°C).
2. While the rising-step mash is underway, make a maltodextrin slurry. While mashing proceeds, the maltodextrin should dissolve in the water. Stir if needed.
3. Add the maltodextrin slurry to the wort and stir to mix in before the beginning of the boil. Boil for 90 minutes, adding hops per schedule, then begin whirlpool.
4. Begin the first whirlpool hop additions once the temperature has reached 170°F (77°C). The temperature will naturally fall to 155°F (68°C), then start second whirlpool hops and hold for 20–30 minutes.
5. After the boil and whirlpool are finished, chill the wort to 70°F (21°C) and pitch yeast.
6. Ferment 10 days at 70°F (21°C), then lower to 60°F (16°C) for a 3-day diacetyl rest after the last dry hop addition.
7. Dry hopping instructions: The first lot of dry hops are added at high krausen, approximately 2 days after active fermentation. Add the second lot of dry hops once the beer has reached final gravity.
8. Carbonate to 2.4 vol. CO_2.

BOOMBASTIC HAZY IPA HOMEBREW
Gluten-Free Hazy IPA

Contributed by Connor Reeves, Holidaily Brewing, Golden, CO

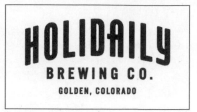

Holidaily Brewing Company was founded in 2016 in Golden, Colorado and is the passion project of founder and chief brewster Karen Hertz, a craft beer enthusiast and lover of living life to the fullest. Karen survived melanoma and thyroid cancers in her early 30s, leading to a treatment plan including a gluten-free diet. Along with beating cancer came the desire to focus on health, happiness, and a commitment to celebrate life every single day.

As a beer lover, being gluten intolerant meant not partaking in social activities in the same way her friends and family could. The lack of good tasting, gluten-free beer options was a challenge Karen was driven to overcome. Years of taste testing gluten-free beers, research on gluten-free ingredients, and an understanding of processes led her to believe there was a better way. And so, the idea of Holidaily Brewing Company was born: a company dedicated to creating world-class gluten-free beer.

Boombastic was Holidaily's first GABF™ Gold Medal winner (2019), and was the inspiration for their canned and distributed Big Henry Hazy IPA—Holidaily's second GABF medal winner.

For 5 US gal. (18.9 L)

Original gravity: 1.059 (14.5°P)
Final gravity: 1.006 (1.5°P)
Color: 4 SRM (8 EBC)

IBU: ~40
ABV: 7%

FERMENTABLES
7.75 lb. (3.25 kg) Grouse pale millet
5.00 lb. (2.27 kg) Grouse pale buckwheat
4.25 lb. (1.98 kg) Grouse Munich millet malt
1.00 lb. (0.45 kg) Grouse flaked quinoa

ENZYMES
18 mL Termamyl® SC DS (equivalent to 1 mL/lb. grain, or 2.2 mL/kg)
27 mL SEBAmyl® L (1.5 mL/lb. grain, or 3.3 mL/kg)

WATER
Adjust for Hazy IPA; suggested levels:
Ca^{2+}: 125–150 ppm, Mg^{2+}: 8 ppm, Na^+ 12 ppm, SO_4^{2-}: 74–100 ppm, Cl^- 175–200 ppm, HCO_3^-: 15 ppm. Acidify sparge water to pH of 6.

BOIL AND WHIRLPOOL HOPS (SEE NOTES)
0.17 oz. (5 g) Citra (12.5% AA) @ 60 min.
0.17 oz. (5 g) Mosaic (12% AA) @ 60 min.
0.17 oz. (5 g) El Dorado (13% AA) @ 60 min.
0.20 oz. (6 g) Citra (12.5% AA) @ whirlpool for 40 min.
0.20 oz. (6 g) Mosaic (12% AA) @ whirlpool for 40 min.
0.20 oz. (6 g) El Dorado (13% AA) @ whirlpool for 40 min.
0.45 oz. (13 g) Citra (12.5% AA) @ whirlpool for 30 min.
0.45 oz. (13 g) Mosaic (12% AA) @ whirlpool for 30 min.
0.45 oz. (13 g) El Dorado (13% AA) @ whirlpool for 30 min.
0.60 oz. (17 g) Citra (12.5% AA) @ whirlpool for 20 min.
0.60 oz. (17 g) Mosaic (12% AA) @ whirlpool for 20 min.
0.60 oz. (17 g) El Dorado (13% AA) @ whirlpool for 20 min.

DRY HOPS

0.65 oz. (18 g) Citra (12.5% AA) dry hop #1 @ high krausen

0.65 oz. (18 g) Mosaic (12% AA) dry hop #1 @ high krausen

0.65 oz. (18 g) El Dorado (13% AA) dry hop #1 @ high krausen

1.00 oz. (28 g) Citra (12.5% AA) dry hop #2 @ 4 days after first dry hop

1.00 oz. (28 g) Mosaic (12% AA) dry hop #2 @ 4 days after first dry hop

1.00 oz. (28 g) El Dorado (13% AA) dry hop #2 @ 4 days after first dry hop

You can substitute the hops for any of your favorites and this recipe will still taste great. This is a basic way to make a Colorado version of a NEIPA. Other hops to consider are Nelson, Sabro, Lotus, Cashmere, Motueka, Paradigm, or other fruit-forward varieties.

YEAST

1 sachet (11.5 g, or 0.4 oz.) Fermentis SafAle™ S-04 dry yeast, or SafAle™ S-33

BREWING NOTES

1. Perform a falling temperature step mash. Mash in using 5.5 gal. (20.8 L) strike water, adding your Termamyl SC DS midway through mashing in. Target the first rest at 175°F (79°C) for 60 minutes. Allow to cool throughout the mash. Once the temperature falls below 165°F (74°C), stir in your SEBAmyl L or other lower-temperature enzymes for a 60-minute second rest.

2. Before the mash is finished, preheat 5.0 gal (18.9 L) sparge water to 195°F (91°C). At the end of the mash, perform your sparge to collect a pre-boil volume of approximately 6.2 gal. (23.5 L).

3. Boil for 60 min., adding boil hops as scheduled. After the boil is complete, cool wort to 180°F (82°C) in the whirlpool before adding first whirlpool hops.

    a. Add first whirlpool hops. After 10 min., add second whirlpool hops. After another 10 min., add third whirlpool hops and let sit in whirlpool for 20 min.

4. When the whirlpool is complete, cool the wort to 72°F (22°C) and transfer to the fermentor. Pitch yeast and ferment at 72°F (22°C) for 10 days, adding dry hops as scheduled.

    a. At high krausen, between 1.022 and 1.014 gravity (5.5°P and 3.5°P), add dry hops #1.

    b. Four days after dry hops #1 were added, add dry hops #2.

5. Four days after dry hops #2 were added, cold crash beer in the fermentor to 32°F (0°C) and condition for 48+ hours, then rack.

6. Carbonate to 2.6 vol. CO_2.

BUCK WILD NEW ZEALAND LAGER
Gluten-Free NZ-Style Lager

Contributed by Buck Wild Brewing Company, Oakland, CA

After adopting a gluten-free diet in 2006, Buck Wild Brewing founder Mike Bernstein's biggest challenge as a craft beer lover was finding a quality beer that was not brewed with barley, wheat, or rye. He figured there had to be a way to brew 100% gluten-free beer that rivaled the high quality and full flavor of today's fantastic craft beers, so he set out to create his own. After many nights and weekends tinkering in his garage and kitchen (along with numerous failed batches), Mike finally brewed a gluten-free beer that friends and family said was actually drinkable (high praise!).

Over the next few years, Mike's homebrews received such glowing reviews that he was inspired to share his beer with a wider audience by bringing it to market. In late 2012, he began collaborating with the beer maestros at UC Davis to focus on improving and scaling his recipes. What started out as a weekend hobby over a decade ago has now become a full-time pursuit and Mike is proud to be at the helm of Buck Wild Brewing.

For 5.5 US gal. (20.8 L)

Original Gravity: 1.051 (12.6 °P)
Final Gravity: 1.009 (2.3°P)
Color: 4 SRM (7 EBC)

IBU: 21
ABV: 5.4%

FERMENTABLES
1.5 lb. (0.68 kg) Eckert pale rice malt
4.0 lb. (1.81 kg) Grouse pale millet malt
1.0 lb. (0.45 kg) Grouse Munich millet malt
2.0 lb. (0.91 kg) Grouse Vienna millet malt
0.5 lb. (0.45 kg) Grouse pale buckwheat malt

ENZYMES
9 mL Termamyl® SC DS (equivalent to 1 mL/lb. grain, or 2.2 mL/kg)
16 mL Ceremix® Flex (1.2 mL/lb. grain, or 2.7 mL/kg)
11 mL Ondea® Pro (1.8 mL/lb. grain, or 4 mL/kg)

WATER
Munich-style water profile; suggested levels:
Ca^{2+}: 75 ppm, Mg^{2+}: 20 ppm, Na^+ 10 ppm, SO_4^{2-}: 10 ppm, Cl^- 2 ppm, HCO_3^-: 200 ppm.

HOPS
0.5 oz. (14 g) Wakatu (3.2% AA) @ 45 min.
1.0 oz. (28 g) Wakatu (3.2% AA) @ 15 min.

YEAST
1 sachet (11.5 g, or 0.4 oz.) Fermentis SafLager™ W-34/70

BREWING NOTES
1. Mash the rice malt first with using the Termamyl SC. Aim for a mash temperature of 190°F (88°C) and rest for 20 min.
2. Mash in the remaining grains to reach 123°F (51°C). Add the Ceremix Flex and Ondea Pro, along with any brewing salts you are using. Rest for 20 min.
3. Raise the mash temperature to 145°F (63°C) and rest for 60 min. Then raise the temperature again to 175°F (79°C) and rest for 20 min.
4. Begin vorlauf until you obtain clear wort. Sparge using 180°F (82°C) water.
5. Boil for 75 min., adding hops as directed. Once the boil is finished, chill the wort to 55°F (13°C).
6. Pitch yeast and ferment at 55°F (13°C) until final gravity is reached.
7. Lager the beer at 45°F (7°C) for 21 days before packaging. Carbonate to 2.7 vol. CO_2.

SMOKED AMBER
Gluten-Free American Amber Ale

Contributed by Robert Keifer

I cannot take any credit for this beer except for the addition of the maple syrup during secondary. All the credit for this beer goes to my wife, Domonic, who designed this recipe in 2019 from what we had on hand at home. There was a special hop we had taken home that year from Homebrew Con™ called Provoak, which we got from hop supplier BarthHaas. Provoak blends both hops and oak together and can be added during secondary to provide a lovely oak-aged taste. This hop paired well with the various roasts Domonic selected. We actually featured the dry hopping of this beer on the YouTube show my wife and I made together, *Baking and Brewing*. This grain bill is a go-to for any amber beer that has a slight touch of smoke to it.

For 5 US gal. (18.9 L)

Original gravity: 1.058 (14.3°P)
Final gravity: 1.012 (3.1°P)
Color: 15–18 SRM (30–36 EBC)

IBU: 20
ABV: 6%

FERMENTABLES

8.00 lb. (3.63 kg) Grouse pale millet malt
1.50 lb. (0.68 kg) Grouse caramel buckwheat
1.00 lb. (0.45 kg) Grouse Dutch Roast millet malt
0.50 lb. (0.23 kg) Grouse Roasted Goldfinch Millet malt
0.50 lb. (0.23 kg) Grouse Red Wing millet malt
0.25 lb. (0.11 kg) cherrywood-smoked rice malt
1.5–3.0 lb. (0.68–1.36 kg) maple syrup – optional, use for secondary fermentation

ENZYMES

12 mL Ceremix® Flex (equivalent to 1.02 mL/lb. grain, or 2.25 mL/kg)
12 mL Ondea® Pro (1.02 mL/lb. grain, or 2.25 mL/kg)

HOPS

2 oz. (57 g) East Kent Goldings (5.3% AA) @ 60 min.

ADDITIONAL ITEMS

1 tablet Whirfloc® @ 15 min.

YEAST

1 package (10 g, or 0.3 oz.) Mangrove Jack's M15 Empire Ale

BREWING NOTES

1. Perform a rising-step mash. Mash in using 4.5 gal. (17 L) strike water to hit 125°F (52°C) and add both enzymes, aiming for 1.0 mL/lb. Rest at 125°F (52°C) for 25 min.
2. Raise mash temperature to 150°F (66°C) and rest for 25 min. Raise mash temperature to 175°F (79°C) and rest for 25 min.
3. Raise temperature to 180°F (82°C) to mash out.
4. Before the mash is finished, preheat sparge water. At the end of the mash out, perform your sparge to collect a pre-boil volume of approximately 6 gal. (22.7 L).
5. When the boil is complete, cool the wort to 68°F (20°C) and transfer to the fermentor.
6. Pitch yeast and ferment at 68°F (20°C) for 14 days.
7. Optional: My favorite version of this beer involves racking it onto maple syrup—let it sit for up to 14 days.
8. Keg and serve. Carbonate to 2.5 vol. CO_2.

INDIA PALE LAGER
Gluten-Free Lager

Contributed by Robert Keifer

The dry hop gives this lager a modern twist, but with a clear tip of the hat to the brewing traditions of central Europe and the British Isles, which appeals to my sense of German and Irish heritage. Since there is a dry hop, I used a lager yeast that produces low levels of diacetyl and favors higher alcohol levels. What's more, this can be fermented at a higher temperature, which will allow for a pleasant aroma on this hoppy lager.

For 5 US gal. (18.9 L)

Original gravity: 1.062 (15.2°P)
Final gravity: 1.011 (2.8°P)
Color: 8–9 SRM (16–18 EBC)

IBU: 35
ABV: 6.7%

FERMENTABLES
6.0 lb. (2.72 kg) Grouse pale millet malt
2.0 lb. (0.91 kg) Eckert biscuit rice malt 4°L
2.0 lb. (0.91 kg) Grouse pale buckwheat malt
1.0 lb. (0.45 kg) Grouse Goldfinch Millet Malt
1.0 lb. (0.45 kg) Eckert amber rice malt
0.5 lb. (0.23 kg) Grouse caramel millet malt 4°L

ENZYMES
13 mL Termamyl® SC DS (equivalent to 1.0 mL/lb. grain, or 2.3 mL/kg)
16 mL SEBAmyl® L (1.3 mL/lb. grain, or 2.8 mL/kg)

HOPS
0.50 oz. (14 g) Hersbrucker (2.3% AA) @ 60 min.
0.75 oz. (21 g) Hallertau Blanc (7.7% AA) @ 30min.
0.50 oz. (14 g) Hersbrucker (2.3% AA) @ 15 min.
0.50 oz. (14 g) Hallertau Blanc (7.7% AA) @ 15 min.
1.00 oz. (28 g) Mandarina Bavaria (8.5% AA) @ dry hop after fermentation
1.00 oz. (28 g) East Kent Goldings (5.6% AA) @ dry hop after fermentation

ADDITIONAL ITEMS
0.5 lb. (0.45 kg) maltodextrin @ 15 min.
½ tablet Whirlfloc® @ 15 min.
0.08 oz. (2.3 g) Yeastex 61 yeast nutrient (allergen warning: contains soy) @ 15 min.

YEAST
1 package (11.5 g, or 0.4 oz.) Fermentis SafLager™ S-189

BREWING NOTES
1. Perform a reverse or falling temperature step mash. Mash in the with all the grains using 22.5 qt. (21.3 L) strike water, targeting a mash temperature of 195°F (91°C). Add the Termamyl SC DS at a rate of 1.0 mL/lb. and rest for 20 min.
2. Recirculate mash liquid to reduce the temperature, or add 1.0 gal. (3.79 L) room-temperature water, to reach 155°F (68°C). Add SEBAmyl L at a rate of 1.25 mL/lb. and rest for 30 min.
3. Vorlauf until wort is clear. Sparge using 2.5–3.0 gal. (9.5–11.4 L) of 209°F (98°C) water, to collect a pre-boil volume of approximately 7 gal. (26.5 L).
4. If you added 1.0 gal. (3.79 L) water in step 2 to bring down the temperature, then adjust your sparge water accordingly, using 1.5–2.0 gal. (5.7–7.6 L).

5. Boil for 60 min., adding hops, maltodextrin, and Whirlfloc as scheduled. Once the boil is finished, chill wort to 55°F (13°C).
6. Pitch yeast at 55°F (13°C) and allow fermentation temperature to rise 1 degree per day for two weeks (roughly 0.5°C/day).
7. Dry hop on day 15 during the diacetyl rest temperature of 68°F (20°C). Let sit for 3 days.
8. Rack to secondary and lager at 35–40°F (2–4°C) for 21 days. Keg and serve carbonated to 2.4 vol. CO_2.

DAD'S RED ALE

Gluten-Free American Red Ale   *Contributed by Joe Morris, founder of Zero Tolerance Gluten Free Homebrew Club*

Joe Morris was gifted his first homebrew kit by his dad. To say thanks, Joe would always make his dad an amber ale or red ale when he would come to visit because that was his preferred style. After Joe went gluten free, getting a similar red hue and chewy malt flavor into a beer proved challenging. Nonetheless, after several attempts at recipe formulation, Joe's gluten-free version won Ground Breaker's 1st Annual Pacific Northwest Gluten-Free Homebrew Competition. The beer went on to score 36 at the National Homebrew Competition and was First Round Winner in the Specialty Beer category. It won a blue ribbon at the Oregon State Fair, again while competing in categories against barley-based beer. It's a tasty beer and, most importantly, Joe's dad loved it.

For 5.5 US gal. (20.8 L)

Original gravity: 1.064 (15.7°P)   **IBU:** 35–45
Final gravity: 1.013 (3.3°P)   **ABV:** 6.7%

FERMENTABLES

10.0 lb. (4.54 kg) Grouse pale millet malt
1.50 lb. (0.68 kg) Grouse Munich millet malt
1.00 lb. (0.45 kg) Grouse roasted Cara Millet malt
0.75 lb. (0.34 kg) Grouse caramel millet malt (3.5-5°L)
0.75 lb. (0.34 kg) Eckert biscuit rice malt

0.75 lb. (0.34 kg) Eckert James' Brown rice malt
0.50 lb. (0.23 kg) Eckert crystal rice malt
0.50 lb. (0.23 kg) Grouse pale buckwheat malt
0.25 lb. (0.11 kg) Grouse chocolate millet malt
0.25 lb. (0.11 kg) Candi Syrup, Inc. D-90™ dark candi syrup – add to the boil

ENZYMES

16 mL Termamyl® SC DS (equivalent to 1 mL/lb. grain, or 2.2 mL/kg)
20 mL SEBAmyl® L (1.25 mL/lb. grain, or 2.75 mL/kg)

HOPS

2 mL hop resin extract* @ 60 min.
0.5 oz. (14 g) Centennial @ 10 min.
0.5 oz. (14 g) Cascade @ 10 min.
0.5 oz. (14 g) Cascade @ whirlpool for 30 min.
0.5 oz. (14 g) Centennial @ whirlpool for 30 min.
0.5 oz. (14 g) Simcoe @ whirlpool for 30 min.
0.5 oz. (14 g) Amarillo @ whirlpool for 30 min.

* This refers to hop resin products extracted using supercritical CO_2. When used as a bittering addition the hop variety is not all that important, so use what you have (the original recipe used CTZ hop extract). If you do not have access to hop extracts like this, use your favorite clean bittering hop and aim for 16 IBU.

YEAST

2 sachets (23 g, or 0.8 oz.) Fermentis SafAle™ S-04

BREWING NOTES

1. Perform a reverse or falling temperature step mash. Mash in the with all the grains using 28.8 qt. (27.3 L) strike water, targeting a mash temperature of 195°F (91°C). Add the Termamyl SC DS at a rate of 1.0 mL/lb. and rest for 20 min.
2. Recirculate mash liquid to reduce the temperature, or add 1.0 gal. (3.79 L) room-temperature water, to reach 155°F (68°C). Add SEBAmyl L at a rate of 1.25 mL/lb. and rest for 30 min.

3. Vorlauf until wort is clear. Sparge using 2.5–3.0 gal. (9.5–11.4 L) water and collect wort into your boil kettle.
   a. If you added 1.0 gal. (3.79 L) water in step 2 to bring down the temperature, then adjust your sparge water accordingly, using 1.5–2.0 gal. (5.7–7.6 L).
4. Boil for 60 min., adding hops and candi syrup at 15 min. Once the boil is finished, chill wort to 68°F (20°C).
5. Pitch yeast and ferment at 68°F (20°C) for 14 days.
6. Cold crash for 3 days. Keg and serve carbonated to 2.5 vol. CO_2.

END GAME IPA

Gluten-Free American IPA

Contributed by Joe Morris, founder of Zero Tolerance Gluten Free Homebrew Club

Joe designed the recipe for this beer before the Marvel movie of the same name. The concept of the beer was to create a beer with a lot of New World hop aroma and flavor. Except for a small bittering charge, all the hops come in the late stages of the brew. Galaxy, Amarillo, Mosaic, and Ekuanot (then Equinox) hops define both the hop profile and the name in this backronym beer.

This beer debuted at Club Night during Homebrew Con™ 2018, where Mike "Tasty" McDole's early support of the club, his praise of this beer, and his presence at the Zero Tolerance booth drew attention to the club's gluten-free offerings. Tasty's approval provided instant legitimacy for Zero Tolerance in traditional brewing circles. Tasty always made time to help brewers and he is dearly missed by all those who knew him.

Batch Size: 6 gal (22.7 L)

Original gravity: 1.068 (16.6°P)
Final gravity: 1.006 (1.005°P)
Color: 5 SRM (10 EBC)

IBU: 86
ABV: 8.1%

FERMENTABLES

10.00 lb. (4.54 kg) Grouse pale millet malt
1.00 lb. (0.45 kg) Grouse caramel millet malt 4°L
0.75 lb. (0.34 kg) Grouse Munich millet malt

5.00 lb. (2.27 kg) Eckert pale rice malt
1.00 lb. (0.45 kg) Belgian candi sugar 0°L –
    add to boil with 15 minutes left

ENZYMES

17 mL Termamyl® SC DS (equivalent to 1.0 mL/lb. grain, or 2.2 mL/kg)
21 mL SEBAmyl® L (1.25 mL/lb. grain, or 2.76 mL/kg)

HOPS

0.1 oz. (3 g) CTZ Extract @ 60 min.
1.0 oz. (28 g) Galaxy (14% AA) @ 5 min.
0.5 oz. (14 g) Amarillo (10% AA) @ 5 min.
1.0 oz. (28 g) Mosaic (12.5% AA) @ 5 min.
0.5 oz. (14 g) Ekuanot (14% AA) @ 5 min.
1.0 oz. (28 g) Amarillo (10% AA) @ whirlpool for 30 min. at 185°F (85°C)
1.0 oz. (28 g) Mosaic (12.5% AA) @ whirlpool for 30 min. at 185°F (85°C)
1.0 oz. (28 g) Galaxy (14% AA) @ whirlpool for 30 min. at 185°F (85°C)
2.0 oz. (57 g) Galaxy (14% AA) @ dry hop for 5 days before cold crash
1.0 oz. (28 g) Amarillo (10% AA) @ dry hop for 5 days before cold crash
1.0 oz. (28 g) Mosaic (12.5% AA) @ dry hop for 5 days before cold crash
0.5 oz. (14 g) Ekuanot (14% AA) @ dry hop for 5 days before cold crash

YEAST

2 sachets (23 g, or 0.8 oz.) Fermentis SafAle™ US-05

BREWING NOTES

1. Perform a reverse or falling temperature step mash. Mash in the with all the grains using 22.05 qt. (20.87 L) strike water, targeting a mash temperature of 195°F (91°C). Add the Termamyl SC DS at a rate of 1.0 mL/lb. and rest for 20 min.
2. Recirculate mash liquid to reduce the temperature, or add 1.0 gal. (3.79 L) room-temperature water, to reach 155°F (68°C). Add SEBAmyl L at a rate of 1.25 mL/lb. and rest for 30 min.

3. Vorlauf until wort is clear, then sparge. You will have to adjust your sparge water volume if you added water in step 2 to bring down the temperature.
4. Boil for 60 min., adding hops and candi sugar as scheduled. Once the boil is finished, chill wort to 68°F (20°C).
5. Pitch yeast and ferment at 68°F (20°C) for 14 days.
6. Cold crash for 3 days. Keg and serve carbonated to 2.5 vol. CO_2.

CHOCOLATE TACO STOUT
Gluten-Free American Stout
Contributed by Ben Fowler

When Ben Fowler (p. 144) was growing up, his favorite treat from the ice cream truck was always Choco Taco®. The waffle cone taco shell has notes of caramel and is filled with vanilla ice cream and then topped with chocolate. Now that he can no longer indulge in gluten, Ben created the next best thing to a Choco Taco: a gluten-free stout with the same flavor profile! Be sure to make your vanilla bean extract in advance of brew day.

For 5.5 US gal. (20.8 L)

Original gravity: 1.068 (16.6°P)
Final gravity: 1.014 (3.6°P)
Color: 29 SRM (57 EBC)

IBU: 61
ABV: 7.7%

FERMENTABLES
8.00 lb. (3.63 kg) Grouse pale millet malt
2.00 lb. (0.91 kg) Grouse pale buckwheat malt
1.50 lb. (0.68 kg) Grouse chocolate roasted millet malt
1.00 lb. (0.45 kg) Grouse light roasted millet malt
1.00 lb. (0.45 kg) Grouse Vienna millet malt
0.75 lb. (0.34 kg) Grouse roasted Cara Millet malt

0.50 lb. (0.23 kg) Grouse Caramel 240L millet malt
0.50 lb. (0.23 kg) Grouse flaked quinoa
0.35 lb. (0.16 kg) Eckert Naked (de-hulled) "Gas Hog" rice malt
2.00 lb. (0.91 kg) rice hulls – to aid in wort separation

ENZYMES
15.6 mL Ceremix® Flex (equivalent to 1.0 mL/lb. grain, or 2.2 mL/kg)
15.6 mL Ondea® Pro (1.0 mL/lb. grain, or 2.2 mL/kg)

HOPS
1.5 oz. (43 g) Centennial (10% AA) @ 60 min.
1.5 oz. (43 g) Cascade (6% AA) @ 15 min.

ADDITIONAL ITEMS
4 tsp (20 mL) Fermaid @ 15 min.
1 tablet Whirfloc® @ 15 min.
cacao and vanilla extract* – to taste in secondary before kegging (Ben uses it all)

YEAST
2 sachets (23 g, or 0.8 oz.) Fermentis SafAle™ US-05

BREWING NOTES
1. Heat strike water to 135°F (57°C) and mash in with entire grist; mash temperature should be 125°F (52°C). Add Ceremix and Ondea Pro and rest for 25 min. at 125°F (52°C).
2. Raise mash to 150°F (66°C) and rest 25 min.
3. Raise mash to 175°F (79°C) and hold for an additional 25 min.
4. Mash out at 180°F (82°C) for 10 min., then perform sparge and boil.
5. Once boil is complete, chill wort to 67°F (19°C), and pitch yeast.
6. Ferment at 67°F (19°C) for 6 days, then cold crash and package.
7. Rack to secondary, add cacao and vanilla extract, and cold crash.
8. Keg and serve carbonated to 2.4 vol. CO_2.

* Cacao and vanilla extract: Split and scrape one vanilla bean and add all parts to 6 fl. oz. (180 mL) unflavored vodka in a sealable glass jar. Shake every day for a week. Add 3 oz. (85 g) of roasted cacao nibs and shake daily for another 4 days. Strain through coffee filter.

SUE'S BREW HAWAIIAN STOUT
Gluten-Free Specialty American Stout   *Contributed by Beliveau Farm*

This beer is named for an old friend of John Hildreth (p. 98), Sue, whose family is Hawaiian and who is also an avid stout enthusiast. The Hawaiian designation obviously comes from the use of Kona coffee, although if you wanted to substitute another variety (e.g., Sumatran or Ethiopian), it would work just as well. The toasted coconut provides a mild burnt caramel bite on the back end of the flavor and doesn't present as coconut (unless you use more of it).

For 5 US gal. (18.9 L)

Original gravity: 1.065 (15.9°P)   **IBU:** 57
Final gravity: 1.018 (4.6°P)   **ABV:** 6.2%
Color: 33 SRM (65 EBC)

FERMENTABLES
7.0 lb. (3.18 kg) Eckert pale rice malt
1.0 lb. (0.45 kg) Grouse Vienna millet malt
1.0 lb. (0.45 kg) Grouse caramel millet malt
   3.5–5°L
0.7 lb. (0.32 kg) Grouse roasted malted buckwheat

0.7 lb. (0.32 kg) Grouse pale buckwheat malt
0.5 lb. (0.23 kg) Eckert dark rice malt
0.5 lb. (0.23 kg) Eckert "Gas Hog" rice malt
1.0 lb. (0.45 kg) Candi Syrup, Inc. D-180™ –
   added in last 10 min. of the boil

ENZYMES
11 mL Ceremix® Flex (equivalent to 0.96 mL/lb. grain, or 2.12 mL/kg)
11 mL Ondea® Pro (0.96 mL/lb. grain, or 2.12 mL/kg)
11 mL Termamyl® (0.96 mL/lb. grain, or 2.12 mL/kg)

WATER
7.60 gal. (28.8 L) distilled water (important for mash pH)
0.30 oz. (9 g) gypsum
0.15 oz. (4.5 g) calcium chloride
0.25 fl. oz. (7.3 mL) lactic acid, 88% solution

HOPS
0.8 oz. (23 g) Willamette (5.5% AA) @ 60 min.
0.8 oz. (23 g) Nugget (13% AA) @ 10 min.
0.8 oz. (23 g) Cluster (7% AA) @ 10 min.

ADDITIONAL INGREDIENTS
4.0 oz. (113 g) tapioca maltodextrin – add before boil starts (see notes)
4.5 oz. (128 g) toasted coconut @ secondary fermentor
4.5 oz. (128 g) rough-ground Kona coffee @ secondary fermentor

YEAST
1 sachet (11.5 g, or 0.4 oz.) Fermentis SafAle™ S-04

BREWING NOTES
1. Use 3.47 gal. (13.14 L) of the water for strike water and reserve the remaining for your fly or batch sparge.
2. Rising-step mash part one: Heat strike water to 135–140°F (57–60°C) and add gypsum and calcium chloride, stirring to dissolve. Add milled grains and stir to mix and evenly distribute the hulls from the rice malts. Add all three enzymes and the lactic acid. Continued >

3. After the mash-in, the mash temperature will be around 130–134°F (54–57°C); mash pH should come in at 5.2–5.3. Mash for 45 minutes, gradually raising the temperature to and holding it at 145°F (63°C).

4. While the rising-step mash is underway, make a maltodextrin slurry. While mashing proceeds, the maltodextrin should dissolve in the water. Stir if needed.

5. Rising-step mash part two: gradually raise mash temperature to 164°F (73°C) over 45 minutes (you can go as high as 170°F, or 77°C). When finished, hold for an additional 15 minutes.

6. Before the mash is finished, preheat sparge water to 180°F (82°C). At the end of the mash, perform your sparge to collect a pre-boil volume of approximately 6 gal. (22.7 L).

7. Add the maltodextrin slurry to the wort and stir to mix in before the beginning of the boil. Boil wort for 60 min., adding hops as scheduled.

8. When the boil is complete, cool the wort and transfer to the fermentor. Pitch yeast and ferment at 64°F (18°C) until specific gravity is stable and fermentation is complete. Rack to a secondary fermentor containing coconut and coffee and let sit for another week.

9. Bottle when ready, allowing two weeks for bottle conditioning before drinking. If kegging, allow the requisite time needed for carbonation to equilibrate. Carbonate to 2.2 vol. CO_2.

Gruit | © Getty/Rosario Scalia

10

Historical Styles

Inspiration for this chapter comes from various styles of beer that are traditionally set within the context of beer's history, both ancient and relatively recent. Many such styles are, in fact, alive and well, albeit some in a different form to their historical namesakes. Those of you who have come up through the conventions of barley brewing in the European tradition may recognize styles like "wee heavy," braggot, and gruit. Beer styles like umqombothi, chicha, and semilla (amaranth beer from Colombia) may not be so recognizable, but are still just as relevant to brewing in historical and present-day contexts. In this chapter, you will see a mix of traditional and modern techniques employed, as befits modern craft brewing's propensity to take inspiration from and reinvent (or reinvigorate) ancient brewing traditions.

There is a chance that some of these brews are more accessible to people outside of the United States and are a much-needed component when creating a book like this. Thank you to all the brewers who contributed recipes to this chapter.

CHICHA
Fermented Maize Beer

Contributed by Dos Luces Brewing, Denver, CO

This recipe is inspired by the traditional fermented or unfermented corn-based beverage consumed for centuries in South and Central America. Either masticated and fermented or sprouted and sun-dried as malt, corn forms the basis of this light and refreshing drink. Chicha (and their agave counterpart, pulque) is commonly blended with fruit, spices, coffee, and chocolate in tantalizing and refreshing combinations.

For 1 US gal. (3.79 L)

Original gravity: 1.055 (13.6°P)
Final gravity: 1.010 (2.6°P)
Color: Purple

IBU: 0
ABV: 5.5–6.0%

FERMENTABLES
2.0 lb. (0.91 kg) malted blue corn
0.5 lb. (0.23 kg) brown sugar or piloncillo* – add during last 15 min. of boil

ENZYMES
2.0 mL Termamyl® SC DS
0.6 mL SacZyme® Pro 1.5X

ADDITIONAL INGREDIENTS
Spices or fruit as you like. One idea: add about ½ tsp of whole cloves for this recipe with 2 cups (0.5 L) of cherry puree.

YEAST
1 sachet (11.5 g, or 0.4 oz.) brewer's yeast, e.g., Fermentis SafAle™ US-05
Pichia† yeast (or substitute with a saison yeast)
Blend yeast strains: For a mixed culture of *Saccharomyces* and *Pichia*, 4 parts *Sacch.* to 1 part *Pichia* works well. Pichia is not readily available so you should plan to substitute with a saison yeast. To make a mixed culture using saison yeast, add half a packet each of Fermentis SafAle™ US-05 and saison yeast strain to the top of the wort you have collected into the fermentation vessel.

BREWING NOTES
1. Perform a reverse or falling step-mash. Mash in all of the corn using 1 gallon, (3.8 L) strike water, targeting a mash temperature of 180°F (82°C). Add Termamyl SC DS at a rate of 1 mL/lb. of corn malt.
2. Drop temperature to 155°F (68°C) for second enzymatic rest. Add the SacZyme Pro 1.5X at a rate of 0.3 mL/lb. corn malt and rest for 30 min.
3. **Boil note:** If you have the capability, perform the boil with the grains. The easiest way to do this is to use a boil-in-a-bag method, making sure the bag is suspended in the boil kettle to prevent the grains or the bag from burning onto the kettle bottom. A kitchen sieve is recommended to strain the grain from the wort if you are not using the BIAB method.
4. Boil wort for 60 min., adding the sugar 10–15 minutes before the end of boil to ensure that it dissolves completely. Once boil is complete, cool wort to at least 75°F (24°C).
5. Pitch your mixed culture (see yeast notes in ingredients). The temperature will vary according to your specific yeast strains, but with a typical mixed culture you would ferment at 72–75°F (22–24°C) for 2–3 weeks.

6. **Serving note:** Chicha is traditionally served while it is fermenting, so you are encouraged to try it frequently during fermentation, and you may even want to drink it "thick" with significant yeast still in solution. There will be some natural carbonation.
7. If packaging, carbonate to 2.6 vol. CO_2.

* Unrefined cane sugar that is commonly used in Mexican cooking. Sometimes called *panela*.
† From the family Saccharomycetaceae, *Pichia* is a genus of yeast often found in chicha and is commercially available through Propagate Lab, CO.

OLD MAN SAGE GRUIT
Gluten-Free Gruit

Contributed By Moonshrimp Brewing, Portland, OR

Brewmaster Dan McIntosh-Tolle advises that this recipe is very sensitive to contamination because it contains no hops at all, so it requires excellent sanitization procedures. Made using a cereal mash, the raw millet will contribute very little to the gravity and so mash efficiency can be ignored. Dan also makes his own invert syrup, caramelizing it until it achieves a deep gold color. The final color of the invert syrup will affect the color of the finished beer, so use the figure below as a rough guide. Be aware that invert syrup caramelized to the point where it goes very dark or black can become bitter.

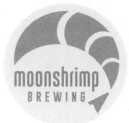

For 5 US gal. (18.9 L)

Original gravity: 1.055 (13.6°P)
Final gravity: 1.010 (2.6°P)

Color: 22 SRM
ABV: 5.5–6.0%

FERMENTABLES
7.0 lb. (3.17 kg) millet seed
5.0 lb. (2.26 kg) invert syrup

1.0 lb. (0.45 kg) honey

ADDITIONAL INGREDIENTS
1.0 oz. (28 g) dry sage leaf (not rubbed sage powder) @ 45 min.
0.5 oz. (14 g) dry orange peel @ 45 min.

YEAST
1 sachet (11.5 g, or 0.4 oz.) Fermentis SafAle™ US-05

BREWING NOTES
1. Grind raw millet before mashing. Mash at a low temperature, strike and sparge at 145°F (63°C).
2. Add the invert syrup to the wort and bring to a boil—do not boil vigorously. Add the sage and orange peel as scheduled; there are no hop additions.
3. After the boil is complete, cover the kettle and let the wort temperature fall to approximately 180°F (82°C) before adding the honey. This preserves more of the honey flavor that would otherwise be lost to boiling. Once the honey is dissolved, cool the wort to 62°F (17°C).
4. Pitch yeast at 62°F (17°C) and let fermentation free rise to 68°F (20°C). The addition of sage slows the fermentation rate, so you should let this ferment for at least 20 days.
5. Once fermentation is over and the gravity is stable, cold crash for 5 days.
6. Carbonate to 2.9 vol CO_2 and package.

UMQOMBOTHI
Traditional Fermented Sorghum Beer

Contributed by Robert Keifer

The moment that I saw Gluten Free Brew Supply was carrying red sorghum malt, the first thought that came to my mind was that I needed to brew a traditional African sorghum beer. I will admit that I used exogenous enzymes the first time I brewed this beer, but this recipe is for anyone, anywhere in the world where malted sorghum is available. This beer is my favorite sour or tart beer that I've ever brewed or tasted. The subtle sauvignon notes that sorghum contributes, with its malty-bitter taste, mixed with tart and funky aroma and flavor notes from the bacteria and the yeast combine to create an incredibly refreshing and easy-sipping beer.

The recipe that follows is a little bit more traditional in that it relies on an overnight sour mash, but the decantation method that is used reflects a more modern approach that understands this malted grain possesses endogenous enzymes. Traditional recipes may involve a longer α-amylase rest (the second rest) and then just a single rise to 180°F (82°C). The decantation method seems to be the best way to ensure the highest starting gravity using malted sorghum grain without resorting to exogenous enzymes.

For 5 US gal. (18.9 L)

Original gravity: 1.055 (13.6°P)	**IBU:** 0
Final gravity: 1.010 (2.6°P)	**ABV:** 5.5–6.0%

FERMENTABLES
8.0 lb. (3.63 kg) red sorghum malt
1.0 lb. (0.45 kg) rice hulls – aids in wort separation

ENZYMES
To brew this beer traditionally requires no exogenous enzymes.

BREWING NOTES
1. Grind the sorghum down to almost a powder. Mix with 4.5 gallons (17 L) 110°F (43°C) water, and slowly raise mash temperature while stirring to 135°F (52°C), then let sit for 30 min.
2. Raise mash to 155°F (68°C) and let sit for another 30 min allowing solids to settle.
3. Decant the liquid off the top of the grains and let sit with cheese cloth covering it.
4. Raise the remainder of the mash to 180°F (82°C) and let sit for 30 min. to gelatinize the grains. Cool to 163°F (73°C). Add back the enzyme-laden liquid you decanted earlier back to the mash and let it sit for 45 min.
5. Heat the whole mash to 180°F (82°C) once again to kill endogenous enzymes. Let the mash cool to 90–100°F (32–38°C), cover with cheese cloth, and let sit overnight to acidify. Overnight, the action of microflora naturally present should lower the mash pH close to 3.8–4.2; if not, let it sit for another 12 hours until it reaches the desired acidity.
6. Heat the mash to 180°F (82°C) and separate the grain from the wort, collecting 6.0 gal. (22.7 L) into the kettle.
   a. If you are mashing using a bag to hold the grains, traditional recipes suggest squeezing the bag to make sure additional grain starches and volatile compounds make it into the boil kettle. This not only provides additional yeast food but, since the beer is consumed during fermentation, this adds to the body as well.
7. Boil the wort for 60 min. There are no boil additions. Once the boil is complete, chill the wort, transfer to a fermentation vessel, cover, and leave. Traditionally, umqombothi is buried in the ground ¾ of the way up the side of the vessel with the opening covered in cheesecloth. It is allowed to ferment for 3–4 days. You can ferment in a regular fermenting bucket or carboy.
8. It is recommended to drink the fermenting beer using a long metal straw to break through the krausen, or head (the bubbly foam layer on top of an actively fermenting beer).

BOCHET BRAGGOT
Gluten-Free Ale Mead with Caramelized Honey
Contributed by Robert Keifer and Evan Mcgann

I brewed this beer back in the summer of 2019 with Evan Mcgann, a member of my local home-brewing club, the OC Mash Ups. Evan typically only brewed mead and cider, so I could actually drink some of the things he would bring to club meetings back when I was a regular attendee. I liked Evan's off-the-wall style, so I had him over to my home brewhouse to brew a braggot, which is today a beer style that often features no hops and is brewed from a half-and-half mix of ale wort and honey. On this particular brew day, I added just enough of a clean bittering hop (Magnum) to balance an otherwise drastically sweet beer.

Evan arrived, honey in hand. He had brought with him relatively light honey (mesquite honey and clover honey) and was talking about a mead style called "bochet," in modern times a name applied to meads originating in Europe that use a technique of boiling down and caramelizing honey into a darker color, thus affecting the color of the resulting mead. These styles of mead can be as black as a stout in fact. Since we were already making a honey-based beer and we had planned on it being more amber in color, I figured why not cook the honeys Evan had brought. The resulting beer was such an amazing experience. Even though it wasn't calculated to be at the usual alcohol level that meads can reach (9%–18% ABV), this beer had an alcoholic warmth to it that suggested it had a higher ABV than the calculated level below. It had a lovely caramelized aroma and burnt marshmallow taste that kept you coming back for a sip time and again. I remember a pretty reckless night of drinking when Evan and I got back together to drink this beverage once it was kegged.

5 US gal. (18.9 L)

Original gravity: 1.065 (15.9°P)
Final gravity: 1.007 (1.8°P)
Color: 12.5 SRM (if you cook the honey longer, you can have an SRM closer to 59)

IBU: 0
ABV: 7.6%

FERMENTABLES
6.00 lb. (2.72 kg) Grouse pale millet malt
2.00 lb. (0.91 kg) Grouse pale buckwheat malt
1.50 lb. (0.68 kg) Eckert crystal rice malt

0.25 lb. (0.11 kg) Grouse caramel C90 millet malt
4.0 lb. (1.81 kg) honey, boiled to make "bochet" – see brewing notes

ENZYMES
9.75 mL Termamyl® SC DS
12.2 mL SEBAmyl® L

HOPS
1.0 oz. (28 g) Magnum (12% AA) @ 30 min.

ADDITIONAL ITEMS
½ tablet Whirfloc® @ 15 min.
1 tbsp yeast nutrient @ 15 min.

YEAST
2 packets (23 g, or 0.8 oz.) Fermentis SafAle™ S-05

BREWING NOTES

1. To make the "bochet": Boil 2.0 lb. (0.91 kg) clover honey and 2.0 lb. (0.91 kg) mesquite honey in two separate sauce pots. You will need two separate spoons for stirring.
   a. Boil the clover honey for 1.5–3 hours until it tastes like burnt marshmallow.
   b. Boil the mesquite honey for 30–60 min. until it has a nice caramel taste.
2. Mash in all the grains using 17.55 qt. (16.6 L) water to achieve a mash temperature of 195°F (91°C). Add the Termamyl SC DS at 1 mL/lb. of grain and rest for 20 min.
3. Recirculate mash liquid, or add 1.0 gal. (3.79 L) of room-temperature water, to drop mash temperature down to 155°F (68°C). Add SEBAmyl L and rest for 30 min.
4. Recirculate until wort is clear. Sparge with 209°F (98.3°C) water, collecting 6.5 gal. (24.6 L) into the boil kettle.
5. Boil for 60 min. Once boil is complete, chill the wort to 68°F (20°C). While wort is chilling, add the bochet.
6. Pitch yeast and ferment at 68°F (20°C) until the airlock is no longer bubbling. Cold crash for 5 days.
7. Package and serve, carbonated to 2.7 vol. CO_2.

HEATHER SCOTCH ALE
Gluten-Free "Wee Heavy"

Contributed by Robert Keifer & Matt Marriott

I brewed this Scotch ale in the fall of 2019 with soon-to-be founder of Suspect Brewing, Matt Marriott. Matt is from Edinburgh and had come to the US to do a gluten-free brewery tour before opening up his own place. Matt has a friend in southern California and, since he was in the area, I invited Matt over to homebrew a Scottish-style ale with gluten-free grains. With a nod to tradition, we added heather tips for a lovely tea-like and spicy note that complemented the resulting high-ABV beer.

This beer was a whopper, seriously. Such a lovely, deep, rich, and complex Scotch ale. The base malt recipe is based on a "wee heavy" recipe that was contributed by Ed Golden to the American Homebrewer's Association, but adjusted to what I had on-hand at the time. This beer is dangerously tasty.

For 5 US gal. (18.9 L)

Original gravity: 1.089 (21.3°P)
Final gravity: 1.010 (2.6°P)
Color: 40

IBU: 10
ABV: 10.37%

FERMENTABLES
10.00 lb. (4.54 kg) Grouse pale millet malt
1.50 lb. (0.68 kg) Eckert biscuit rice malt 4°L
1.00 lb. (0.45 kg) Grouse Red Wing millet malt
0.50 lb. (0.23 kg) Grouse roast buckwheat, unmalted
0.50 lb. (0.23 kg) Grouse chocolate millet malt
0.25 lb. (0.11 kg) Eckert Pitch Black rice malt
3.30 lb. (1.50 kg) BriesSweet™ White Sorghum Extract
2.00 lb. (0.91 kg) Candi Syrup, Inc. D-45™ dark amber candi syrup

ENZYMES
15 mL Ondea® Pro (1.1 mL/lb.)
15 mL Ceremix® Flex (1.1 mL/lb.)

ADDITIONAL INGREDIENTS
2 oz. (57 g) heather tips @ whirlpool for 30 min.

YEAST
3 sachets (30 g, or 0.9 oz.) Mangrove Jack's M15 Empire Ale

BREWING NOTES
1. Perform a rising temperature step mash. Use 5.5 gal. (20.8 L) strike water and mash in with whole grain bill plus the Ondea Pro and Ceremix Flex. Target a mash temperature of 125°F (52°C) and rest 15 min.
2. Raise mash temperature to 145°F (63°C) and rest 60 min.
3. Raise mash temperature to 175°F (79°C) and rest 60 min.
4. Use 3.0 gal. (11.4 L) at 180°F (82°C) to sparge, collecting 7.5 gal. (28.4 L) into the boil kettle.
5. Boil for 90 min. At the end of the boil, add the heather tips and whirlpool for 30 min. After the whirlpool, cool wort to 68°F (20°C).
6. Pitch yeast and ferment at 68°F (20°C) for up to 4 weeks or until fermentation is complete.
7. Cold crash and package. Carbonate to 2.4 vol. CO_2.

SEMILLA
South American Amaranth Beer

Contributed by Luis Miguel Obando Tobon

The inspiration behind Semilla was Luis' desire to highlight the process and care that Andean grains like quinoa and amaranth need during the growing season to be prime for making gluten-free beer: plowing the land, sowing, watching the seeds grow, then collecting and germinating them for malting. There are no companies that offer malted quinoa and amaranth so most of the time the indigenous communities of South America malt their own.

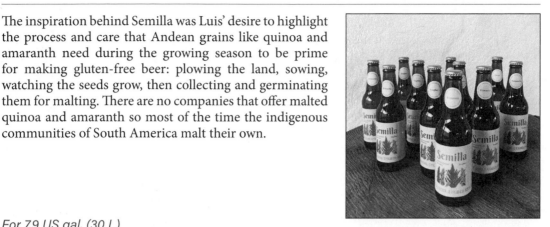

For 7.9 US gal. (30 L)

Boil: 60 minutes + 20 minute WP
Original gravity: 1.040 (10°P)
Final gravity: 1.012 (3.1°P)

Color: 3
IBU: 9
ABV: 3.6%

FERMENTABLES
8.1 lb. (4.0 kg) malted amaranth
14 oz. (0.4 kg) coffee husks – aids in wort separation; alternatively, substitute 0.5 lb. (0.23 kg) rice hulls

ENZYMES
17.1 mL Ceremix® Flex
8.5 mL Ondea® Pro

HOPS
0.6 oz (17 g) Northern Brewer @ 60 min.
0.5 oz (14 g) East Kent Golding @ whirlpool for 20 min. at 190°F (88°C)
0.4 oz (12 g) Fuggle @ whirlpool for 20 min. at 190°F (88°C)

ADDITIONAL ITEMS
1 tablet Whirfloc® @ 15 min.

YEAST
Safale S-04 (Fermentis)

BREWING NOTES
1. Mash in with all the grain into 3.7 gal. (14.0 L) of 127°F (53°C) water, add both enzymes, and rest for 20 minutes. Mash pH should be 5.2–5.4.
2. Raise mash temperature to 144°F (62°C) and rest for 60 min.
3. Raise mash temperature to 175°F (79°C) and rest for 30 min.
4. Sparge using 176°F (80°C) water. Collect 9.25 gal. (35 L) into boil kettle.
5. Boil for 60 min., adding hops and whirlfloc as scheduled. After boil and whirlpool are complete, cool wort to 65°F (18°C).
6. Pitch yeast and ferment for 5 days at 65°F (18°C), then continue fermenting at 70°F (21°C) for a further 7 days.
7. Cold crash for 5 days prior to packaging. Carbonate to 2.6 vol. CO_2.

Appendix A

There's a hole in my assay, dear ELISA, dear ELISA!

Using MS to detect hydrolysed gluten
that is responsible for false negatives by ELISA

Michelle L. Colgrave[1], Harry Goswami[1], Crispin Howitt[2] & Greg Tanner[2].

CSIRO AGRICULTURE & FOOD
www.csiro.au

Gluten is the collective name for a class of proteins found in wheat, rye, barley and oats. Eating gluten triggers an inappropriate autoimmune reaction in ~70 million people globally affected by coeliac disease (CD). In CD the gut reacts to gluten proteins and this triggers an immune response, resulting in intestinal inflammation and damage. Gluten free foods are now commonplace, however, it is difficult to accurately determine the gluten content of products claiming to be gluten-free using current methodologies as the antibodies are nonspecific, show cross-reactivity and have different affinities for the different classes of gluten. The measurement of gluten in processed products is further confounded by modifications to the proteins that occur during processing and in some cases hydrolysis of the proteins.

1   CSIRO Agriculture & Food, St Lucia QLD 4067, Australia.
2   CSIRO Agriculture & Food, Canberra, ACT 2601, Australia.

RESULTS

LC-MS/MS analysis of barley-derived beers revealed that certain classes of hordein were prone to hydrolysis (B- and D-hordein). The resulting peptide fragments shared significant homology with the immunotoxic epitopes determined for CD. Strikingly, those beers that contained high levels of B-hordein fragments gave near zero values by ELISA. The hydrolysed fragments that persist in beer show a dose-dependent suppression of ELISA measurement of gluten despite using a hordein standard for calibration of the assay.

PROTEOMIC PROFILING OF SIZE-FRACTIONATED BEER REVEALS GLUTEN HYDROLYSIS PRODUCTS

GLUTEN	HYDROLYSED
B1-hordein	$57 \pm 12\%$
B3-hordein	$37 \pm 7\%$
D-hordein	$31 \pm 13\%$
γ3-hordein	$18 \pm 10\%$

LC-MS/MS analysis of 60 commercial beers was undertaken after: (1) no filtration (trypsin digestion); (2) <30 kDa filtration (trypsin digestion); or (3) <10 kDa filtration (no digestion).

- Significant hydrolysis of hordeins (gluten) occurred during brewing. Some classes of gluten were more prone to hydrolysis (judged by levels in the <30 kDa fraction relative to whole beer):
- Gluten fragments detected in the sub-10 kDa fraction contained epitopes that would likely be recognised by the antibodies used in currently accepted ELISA technology:
  - → The Skerritt antibody recognises QQGYYP
  - → The Mendez R5 antibody recognises **QQPFP**, QQQFP, LQPFP & QLPFP
- Typical examples of gluten hydrolysis fragments detected include:
  - → B1-hordein (Uniprot: P06470 and I6SJ22) peptide fragments QPQPYP**QQPFP**PQ and P**QQPFP**QQPPFG
- QPQPY**QQPFP**PQ shares 6/9 in the DQ8 T-cell epitope(EQ**QQPFP**Q) and P**QQPFP**QQP PFG shares 8/9 residues in the DQ2 T-cell epitope(**QQPFP**EQPQ) rendering them likely to possess immunoreactivity.

Table 1. Potential immunoreactive peptide sequences. Peptide sequences identified (>95% confidence) in the sub-10 kDa fraction of 60 commercial beers. The sequences are aligned with the closest matching immunoreactive epitope(s). Glutamic acid residues shown in bold typefont(**E**) are produced by deamidation of glutamine (Q) by the enzyme tissue transglutaminase, but are present as Q in the native protein.

PROTEIN NAME	UNIPROT	PEPTIDE SEQUENCE	IMMUNOREACTIVE EPITOPE	# AA MATCHING
B1-hordein	I6TMW0	QPQPYPQQPQQPFPPQ	QQPEQPFPQ	8/9
B1-hordein	P06470	QPQPYPQQPFPPQ	QQPEQPFPQ	6/9
B1-hordein	I6SJ22	PQQPFPQQPPFG	QQPFPEQPQ	8/9
B3-hordein	I6SW30	QPQPYPQQPQPFPQ	PYPEQEQPF	8/9
C-hordein	Q40055	PQPQQPNPQQPQQP	QQPEQPYPQ	6/9
HMW glutenin	J3S7U9	GQGQSGYYPTSPQQP	QGYYPTSPQ	8/9
HMW glutenin	C8CHI1	TSPQQGQQGQQGYYPTSPQQSGQWQ	QGYYPTSPQ	9/9
75k γ-secalin	E5KZU9	PQQPQQSSPQPQQP	PQPEQPFPW	6/9
γ-prolamin	H8Y0J7	GQGIIQPQQPAQLEAIR	IQPEQPAQL	9/9
γ-prolamin	H8Y0J7	QPQQQPPFPQPSQP	PFPQPEQPF	7/9
γ-gliadin	J7HY97	IIQPQQPAQLEVLR	IQPEQPAQL	9/9
γ-gliadin	F6KV50	PQQPQQPAQLEGIR	IQPEQPAQL	8/9
LMW glutenin	G0YLZ2	QQQPFPQQPP	QQPFPEQPQ	8/9
γ-gliadin	L7R5Y9	FPQPQQTIPHQPQ	PFPQPEQPF	6/9
γ-gliadin	B6DQC6	IIQPQQPAQLEVIR	IQPEQPAQL	9/9

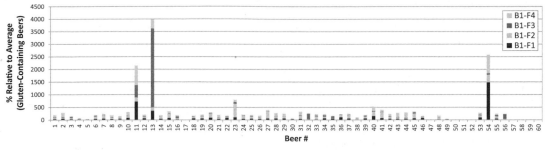

Figure 1. Multiple reaction monitoring (MRM) mass spectrometry reveals gluten fragments in <10 kDa fraction of beers. B-hordein derived peptides B1-F1 through B1-F4 were detected in high levels in beers 11, 13 and 54. These peptide fragments contained the Skerritt or Skerritt-like epitopes.

ELISA RESPONSE IS SUPPRESSED BY HYDROLYSED GLUTEN

- The ELISA Systems assay (Skerritt antibody) is a sandwich ELISA that measures the amount of antigen between a capture and a detection antibody, thus the antigen must have >2 binding sites.
- The hydrolysed gluten fragments present in beer 13 have one potential antigenic site. It was hypothesised that their binding to the capture antibody precludes the binding of intact gluten proteins resulting in suppression of the ELISA response.
- Beer 13 showed a concentration-dependent suppression of the ELISA response (Fig. 2) that was demonstrated to be due primarily to the <3kDa fraction, i.e. hydrolysed peptide fragments. Suppression was also caused by the high MW fraction (30-100 kDa) possibly the result of aggregation (Fig. 3).

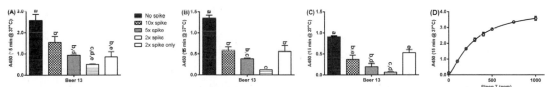

Figure 2. Suppression of ELISA response by hydrolysed gluten present in whole beer. Beer 13 (that contained high levels of hydrolysed gluten) was spiked into samples of beers with differing levels of total gluten: (A) beer 6 (high); (B) beer 31 (medium); and (C) beer 44 (low). The columns represent (from left to right) no spike, spike with diluted beers (at either 10-, 5-or 2-fold dilutions) or the 2-fold diluted spike only. The mean A450 ±SE are shown. The standard curve for calibrating the ELISA assay is shown in panel (D). Two-dimensional analysis of variance (ANOVA) was carried out for each beer (GraphPAD Prism 6.03). Overall p-values were $p \leq 0.0013$ (Beer 6), $p \leq 0.003$ (Beer 31), and $p \leq 0.0001$ (Beer 44). Within a group, columns with different letters were significantly different by Tukey's multiple comparison test ($p \leq 0.01$).

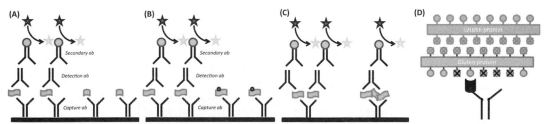

Figure 3. Signal suppression in a sandwich ELISA. In a sandwich ELISA, the capture antibody is bound to the ELISA plate and binds the antigen. The detection antibody binds the antigen at a second site. Gluten proteins contain multiple binding sites. Enzyme-linked secondary antibodies are added and bind to the detection antibody. Finally, the substrate is added, and is converted by the enzyme to a detectable form. (A) Hydrolysed gluten proteins that contain only a single antibody binding site that are present in beer may saturate the capture antibody and suppress the ELISA response. (B) Modifications to the protein that occur during processing may mask binding sites. (C) Aggregation of proteins may sterically hinder binding of the antigen to the capture antibody or the detection antibody to the antigen. (D) As gluten proteins contain multiple binding sites, the model is further complicated. The binding of a single epitope to the antibody may preclude binding at neighbouring epitopes (black crosses). Moreover, protein aggregation may preclude binding in the regions of protein-protein interaction (grey crosses).

CONCLUSIONS

The development of MS-based methodology for absolute quantification of gluten is required for the accurate assessment of gluten, including hydrolysed forms, in food and beverages to support the industry, legislation and to protect consumers suffering from coeliac disease.

References

Colgrave, M.L., Goswami, H., Blundell, M., Howitt, C.A. & Tanner, G.J. (2014) Using mass spectrometry to detect hydrolysed gluten that is responsible for false negatives by ELISA. *Journal of Chromatography* A, 1370, 105-114

Acknowledgments

The authors would like to thank Mr. Alun Jones and the Molecular and Cellular Mass Spectrometry Facility at the University of Queensland for access to the mass spectrometry facility used in this study.

This poster reprinted and used by permission.

Bibliography

Akeroyd, M., S. van Zandycke, J. den Hartog, J. Mutsaers, L. Edens, M. van den Berg, and C. Christis. 2016. "AN-PEP, Proline-Specific Endopeptidase, Degrades All Known Immunostimulatory Gluten Peptides in Beer Made from Barley Malt." *Journal of the American Society of Brewing Chemists* 74(2): 91–99. https://doi.org/10.1094/ASBCJ-2016-2300-01.

Alcohol and Tobacco Tax and Trade Bureau. 2008. "Classification of Brewed Products as 'Beer' Under the Internal Revenue Code of 1986 and as 'Malt Beverages' Under the Federal Alcohol Administration Act." TTB Ruling 2008-03, July 7, 2008. www.ttb.gov/images/pdfs/rulings/2008-3.pdf.

Allred, L. K., K. Lesko, D. McKiernan, C. Kupper, and S. Guandalini. 2017. "The Celiac Patient Antibody Response to Conventional and Gluten-Removed Beer." *Journal of AOAC INTERNATIONAL* 100(2): 485–491. https://doi.org/10.5740/jaoacint.16-0184.

Boz, H. 2015. "Ferulic Acid in Cereals – a Review." *Czech Journal of Food Sciences* 33:1–7.

Bruwer. "Making Umqumbothi to Turn It into Whiskey, Will It Work? Part 1 (The Wash)." Beaver DIY. Uploaded July 12, 2020. YouTube video, 21:28. www.youtube.com/watch?v =Kd7qmQqUZFM&t=970s.

Caio, G., U. Volta, A. Sapone, D. A. Leffler, R. De Giorgio, C. Catassi, and A. Fasano. 2019. "Celiac Disease: A Comprehensive Current Review." *BMC Medicine* 17:142. https://doi.org/10.1186 /s12916-019-1380-z.

Cebolla, Á., M. de Lourdes Moreno, L. Coto, and C. Sousa. 2018. "Gluten Immunogenic Peptides as Standard for the Evaluation of Potential Harmful Prolamin Content in Food and Human Specimen." *Nutrients* 10(12): 1927. https://doi.org/10.3390/nu10121927.

Cleveland Clinic. "Celiac Disease." Updated January 10, 2020. https://my.clevelandclinic.org/health /diseases/14240-celiac-disease.

Colgrave, M. L., H. Goswami, C. A. Howitt, and G. J. Tanner. 2012. "What Is in a Beer? Proteomic Characterization and Relative Quantification of Hordein (Gluten) in Beer." *Journal of Proteome Research* 11(1): 386–396. https://doi.org/10.1021/pr2008434.

Colgrave, M. L., H. Goswami, M. Blundell, C. A. Howitt, and G. J. Tanner. 2014. "Using Mass Spectrometry to Detect Hydrolysed Gluten in Beer That Is Responsible for False Negatives by ELISA." *Journal of Chromatography A* 1370:105–114. https://doi.org/10.1016 /j.chroma.2014.10.033.

Colgrave, M. L., K. Byrne, M. Blundell, and C. A. Howitt. 2016. "Identification of Barley-Specific Peptide Markers That Persist in Processed Foods and Are Capable of Detecting Barley Contamination by LC-MS/MS." *Journal of Proteomics* 147:169–176. https://doi.org/10.1016/j. jprot.2016.03.045.

Colgrave, M. L., K. Byrne, and C. A. Howitt. 2017. "Liquid Chromatography–Mass Spectrometry Analysis Reveals Hydrolyzed Gluten in Beers Crafted To Remove Gluten." *Journal of Agricultural and Food Chemistry* 65(44): 9715–9725. https://doi.org/10.1021/acs.jafc.7b03742.

Cooper, Raymond. 2015. "Re-Discovering Ancient Wheat Varieties as Functional Foods." *Journal of Traditional and Complementary Medicine* 5(3): 138–143. https://doi.org/10.1016/j.jtcme .2015.02.004.

Corne, Lucy. "Embracing Tradition — To Create a Style for the Future, South African Brewers Look to the Past." *Good Beer Hunting*, 11 June 2020. https://www.goodbeerhunting.com/blog/2020/6/9 /embracing-tradition-to-create-a-style-for-the-future-south-african-brewers-look-to-the-past.

Daly, M., S. N. Bromilow, C. Nitride, P. R. Shewry, L. A. Gethings, and E. N. Clare Mills. 2020. "Mapping Coeliac Toxic Motifs in the Prolamin Seed Storage Proteins of Barley, Rye, and Oats Using a Curated Sequence Database." *Frontiers in Nutrition* 7:87. https://doi.org/10.3389 /fnut.2020.00087.

Fasano, A., and C. Catassi. 2001. "Current Approaches to Diagnosis and Treatment of Celiac Disease: An Evolving Spectrum." *Gastroenterology* 120(3): 636–651. https://doi.org/10.1053 /gast.2001.22123.

Gasbarrini, G. B., F. Mangiola, V. Gerardi, G. Ianiro, G. R. Corazza, and A. Gasbarrini. 2014. "Coeliac Disease: An Old or a New Disease? History of a Pathology." *Internal and Emergency Medicine* 9:249–256. https://doi.org/10.1007/s11739-013-1044-5.

Hardy, M. Y., J. A. Tye-Din, J. A. Stewart, F. Schmitz, N. L. Dudek, I. Hanchapola, A. W. Purcell, R. P. Anderson. 2015. "Ingestion of Oats and Barley in Patients with Celiac Disease Mobilizes Cross-Reactive T Cells Activated by Avenin Peptides and Immuno-dominant Hordein Peptides." *Journal of Autoimmunity* 56:56–65. https://doi.org/10.1016/j.jaut.2014.10.003.

Jin, Y-L., R. A. Speers, A. T. Paulson, and R. J. Stewart. 2004. "Barley beta-Glucans and Their Degradation During Malting and Brewing." *Master Brewers Association of the Americas Technical Quarterly* 41(3): 231–240.

Kerau, Mee. "Making Omalovu Giilya 101 | Ft Mee Kerau | Owambo Traditional beer." Its Pero. Uploaded October 25, 2020. YouTube video, 6:14. https://www.youtube.com /watch?v=hVuL4Lb74pg.

Knezevic, J., C. Starchl, A. T. Berisha, and K. Amrein. 2020. "Thyroid-Gut-Axis: How Does the Microbiota Influence Thyroid Function?" *Nutrients* 12(6): 1769. https://doi.org/10.3390 /nu12061769.

Kowalski, K., A. Mulak, M. Jasińska, and L. Paradowski. 2017. "Diagnostic Challenges in Celiac Disease." *Advances in Clinical and Experimental Medicine* 26(4): 729–737. https:// doi.org/10.17219/acem/62452.

Krysiak, R., W. Szkróbka, and B. Okopień. 2019. "The Effect of Gluten-Free Diet on Thyroid Autoimmunity in Drug-Naïve Women with Hashimoto's Thyroiditis: A Pilot Study." *Experimental and Clinical Endocrinology and Diabetes* 127(7): 417–422. https://doi.org/10.1055/a-0653-7108.

Ledley, A. J., R. J. Elias, H. Hopfer, and D. W. Cockburn. 2021. "A Modified Brewing Procedure Informed by the Enzymatic Profiles of Gluten-Free Malts Significantly Improves Fermentable Sugar Generation in Gluten-Free Brewing." *Beverages* 7(3): 53. https://doi.org/10.3390 /beverages7030053.

Lempie and Ale. "HOW TO BREW TRADITIONAL BEER- VILLAGE LIFE IN OWAMBOLAND NAMIBIA- Lempies." Lempies. Uploaded June 15, 2019. YouTube video, 10:37. www.youtube .com/watch?v=bCVwUY5aaj0.

Lerner, A., P. Jeremias, and T. Matthias. 2017. "Gut-Thyroid Axis and Celiac Disease." *Endocrine Connections* 6(4): R52–R58. https://doi.org/10.1530/ec-17-0021.

Lincoln, Anda. "Africa, traditional brewing in,." Oxford Companion to Beer definition of. *Craft Beer & Brewing*. https://beerandbrewing.com/dictionary/izd8yFIQEc/.

Lopez, M., and L. Edens. 2005. "Effective Prevention of Chill-Haze in Beer Using an Acid Proline-Specific Endoprotease from *Aspergillus niger*." *Journal of Agricultural and Food Chemistry* 53(20): 7944–7949. https://doi.org/10.1021/jf0506535.

Lucia, S. M., C. Marius, C. Aldea, S. Genel, and F. Emanuela. 2018. "Celiac Disease a Road Paved with Many Obstacles. Differential Diagnosis in Children." *International Journal of Celiac Disease* 6(1): 7–10. https://doi.org/10.12691/ijcd-6-1-5.

Mahadov, S., and P. H. R. Green. 2011. "Celiac Disease: A Challenge for All Physicians." *Gastroenterology and Hepatology (N Y)* 7(8): 554–556.

MBAA. 2018. "Minimum Good Brewing Practices for the U.S. Brewing Industry." HACCP — Food Safety Decision Guide for the Brewing Industry [web page]. Supporting Documents. Master Brewers Association of the Americas Food Safety Committee, April 25, 2018. https:// www.mbaa.com/brewresources/foodsafety/haccp/Documents /MBAAGoodBrewingPractices25April2018.docx.

Niro, S., A. D'Agostino, A. Fratianni, L. Cinquanta, and G. Panfili. 2019. "Gluten-Free Alternative Grains: Nutritional Evaluation and Bioactive Compounds." *Foods* 8(6): 208. https://doi.org /10.3390/foods8060208.

Palmer, John J. 2017. *How to Brew: Everything You Need to Know to Brew Great Beer Every Time.* 4th ed. Boulder, CO: Brewers Publications.

Palmer, John J., and Colin Kaminski. 2012. *Water: A Comprehensive Guide for Brewers.* Boulder, CO: Brewers Publications.

Popp, A., and M. Mäki. 2019. "Gluten-Induced Extra-Intestinal Manifestations in Potential Celiac Disease—Celiac Trait." *Nutrients* 11(2): 320. https://doi.org/10.3390/nu11020320.

Pruimboom, L., and K. de Punder. 2015. "The Opioid Effects of Gluten Exorphins: Asymptomatic Celiac Disease." *Journal of Health, Population and Nutrition* 33:24. https://doi.org/10.1186/s41043-015-0032-y.

Roy, Christopher. "Brewing Milet Beer in Africa." Uploaded January 27, 2017. YouTube video, 33:15. www.youtube.com/watch?v=LMQFoQES3Ho.

Rzychon, M., M. Brohée, F. Cordeiro, R. Haraszi, F. Ulberth, and G. O'Connor. 2017. "The feasibility of harmonizing gluten ELISA measurements." *Food Chemistry* 234:144–154. https://doi.org/10.1016/j.foodchem.2017.04.092.

Sasso F. C., O. Carbonara, R. Torella, A. Mezzogiorno, V. Esposito, L. deMagistris, M. Secondulfo, R. Carratu, D. Iafusco, and M. Cartenì. 2004. "Ultrastructural Changes in Enterocytes in Subjects with Hashimoto's Thyroiditis." *Gut* 53(12): 1878–1880. https://dx.doi.org/10.1136/gut.2004.047498.

Scherf, K.A., A-C. Lindenau, L. Valentini, M. Carmen Collado, I. García-Mantrana, M. Christensen, D. Tomsitz, C. Kugler, T. Biedermann, and K. Brockow. 2019. "Cofactors of Wheat-Dependent Exercise-Induced Anaphylaxis Do Not Increase Highly Individual Gliadin Absorption in Healthy Volunteers." *Clinical and Translational Allergy* 9:19. https://doi.org/10.1186/s13601-019-0260-0.

Stewart, Graham G. "free amino nitrogen (FAN)." Oxford Companion to Beer definition of. *Craft Beer & Brewing.* https://beerandbrewing.com/dictionary/o1j9KOtQ4v/.

Syage, J. A., C. P. Kelly, M. A. Dickason, A. Cebolla Ramirez, F. Leon, R. Dominguez, and J. A. Sealey-Voyksner. 2018. "Determination of Gluten Consumption in Celiac Disease Patients on a Gluten-Free Diet." *American Journal of Clinical Nutrition* 107(2): 201–207. https://doi.org/10.1093/ajcn/nqx049.

Tanner, G. J., M. L. Colgrave, M. J. Blundell, H. P. Goswami, and C. A. Howitt. 2013. "Measuring Hordein (Gluten) in Beer – A Comparison of ELISA and Mass Spectrometry." *PLoS ONE* 8(2): e56452. https://doi.org/10.1371/journal.pone.0056452.

Tonsmeire, Michael. 2014. *American Sour Beers: Innovative Techniques for Mixed Fermentations.* Boulder: Brewers Publications.

Wieser, Herbert, Peter Koehler, and Katharina Konitzer. 2014. *Celiac Disease and Gluten: Multidisciplinary Challenges and Opportunities.* London: Academic Press.

Zarnkow, M., M. Keßler, W. Back, E. K. Arendt, and M. Gastl. 2010. "Optimisation of the Mashing Procedure for 100% Malted Proso Millet (*Panicum miliaceum* L.) as a Raw Material for Gluten-Free Beverages and Beers." *Journal of the Institute of Brewing* 116(2): 141–150. https://doi.org /10.1002/j.2050-0416.2010.tb00410.x.

INDEX